OXFORD MEDICAL

Talking with Patients

Talking with Patients
A Basic Clinical Skill

PHILIP R. MYERSCOUGH
Deputy Chief of Services (Obstetrics and Gynaecology)
Sultanate of Oman

With Contributions by

A. L. SPEIRS
former Consultant Paediatrician, Royal Hospital for
Sick Children, Glasgow

R. M. WRATE
Consultant in Adolescent Psychiatry, University
of Edinburgh

C. T. CURRIE
Senior Lecturer in Geriatric Medicine, University
of Edinburgh

D. DOYLE
Medical Director, St Columba's Hospice,
Edinburgh

OXFORD   NEW YORK   TOKYO
OXFORD UNIVERSITY PRESS
1989

Oxford University Press, Walton Street, Oxford OX2 6DP

Oxford   New York   Toronto
Delhi   Bombay   Calcutta   Madras   Karachi
Petaling Jaya   Singapore   Hong Kong   Tokyo
Nairobi   Dar es Salaam   Cape Town
Melbourne   Auckland

and associated companies in
Berlin   Ibadan

Oxford is a trade mark of Oxford University Press

Published in the United States
by Oxford University Press, New York

British Library Cataloguing in Publication Data
Myerscough P. R. (Philip Roger),
Talking with patients
1. Doctors. Communication with patients
I. Title
610.69'6
ISBN 0-19-261769-9

Library of Congress Cataloging-in-Publication Data
Myerscough, P. R. (Philip Roger)
Talking with patients : a basic clinical skill / Philip R.
Myerscough ; with contributions by A.L. Spiers . . . [et al.].
(Oxford medical publications)
Bibliography   Includes index.
1. Physician and patient.   2. Medical personnel and patient.
3. Interpersonal communication.   I. Title.   II. Series.
[DNLM: 1. Communication.   2. Physician-Patient Relations.   W 62
M9963t]
R727.3.M94   1989   610.69'6—dc 19   89-2930
ISBN 0-19-261769-9

Set by Downdell Limited
Printed in Great Britain
by Biddles Ltd.
Guildford & King's Lynn

Preface

This book has been written primarily for medical students who are embarking on clinical work. It will also be helpful reading for senior students and young doctors who are aiming to improve their communication skills and so to prepare a sound foundation for a career in any branch of clinical medicine. The author and his contributors have endeavoured to set out in a clear and concise manner the elements that promote good communication, and the skills through which these are deployed in day-to-day practice.

This area of learning is of equal importance for students of nursing, and of other health professions, particularly those whose work involves touching as well as talking. It is not assumed that the reader already has any great depth of knowledge of either clinical or behavioural science. Although the focus of the volume is on the verbal interaction between patient and doctor—the medical interview—the skills described can readily be applied in other professional settings.

As well as interpersonal dialogue, other dimensions of communication are discussed, including written communication. A recurring theme throughout the book is the manner in which the doctor (or other health professional) can facilitate or, regrettably, inhibit the expression by the patient of the feelings and concerns that are likely to arise during illness.

The need for medical training to include greater emphasis on communication skills is now becoming widely recognized. The Education Committee of the General Medical Council underlined this need in its Recommendations (1980), and made communication the topic of its annual educational symposium in 1987. The Royal College of Physicians of London has given notice that assessment of communication skills will in future form part of the Membership examination. The Royal College of Physicians of Edinburgh has recently promoted a major symposium on this topic. From the other side of the fence, the Patients Association and other groups representing clients regularly express their concern that doctors and other health professionals should learn to communicate better.

In most of the text both the patient and the doctor are referred to as 'he' rather than the more cumbersome 'he or she' in every instance. This in no way implies any intention of devaluing the female sex, or ignoring the role of women in medicine. It is merely a convenience of style.

I am greatly indebted to the four colleagues who have each contributed a chapter in their own areas of special expertise. This has brought to the book a breadth and diversity that it would not otherwise have achieved. They are:

Dr A.L. Speirs, *OBE, MD, FRCP (London and Glasgow), DCH, former Consultant Paediatrician, Royal Hospital for Sick Children, Glasgow, Stirling Royal Infirmary, and Falkirk and District Royal Infirmary.*

Dr R.M. Wrate, *DPM, FRC Psych, Consultant in Adolescent Psychiatry. Hon. Senior Lecturer, Department of Psychiatry, University of Edinburgh.*

Dr C.T. Currie, *FRCP Ed, Senior Lecturer in Geriatric Medicine, University of Edinburgh.*

Dr D. Doyle, *OBE, FRCS Ed, FRCP Ed, FRCGP, Medical Director, St Columba's Hospice, Edinburgh.*

My thanks are also due to my former departmental colleague Dr Tony Bramley, who provided the line drawings.

Oman   P.R.M.
June 1988

Contents

1 Introduction

Most medical students approach their training with a desire to help people. Thus, from the very beginning of their studies, students look forward to clinical involvement—to meeting 'real' patients and learning to interact with them. After qualifying, most doctors spend a great deal of their working time communicating with patients—speaking, listening, responding. This face-to-face interaction, with exchange of information, is essential if the doctor is to be effective in his or her work.

Accordingly, skilful communication has become widely recognized as a primary component of medical education, something that the student should learn about as a basic part of professional training. However, this is the very aspect of doctors' professional skills that is still the most common cause of complaint from patients or their relatives, an apparent weak point in doctors' professional competence [1,9,10,11,12,13].

Patients particularly single out the affective dimensions of communication as unsatisfactory: doctors are regarded as people with whom it is often difficult to talk about the feelings associated with illness. Conversely, patients' feelings of satisfaction after consultations relate to the doctor's friendliness, his understanding of their expectations, and his ability to cope with their worries and concerns [2,3,4].

Only recently have formal attempts been made to teach communication skills to medical students in Britain. These efforts are usually scattered about the curriculum, are fairly limited in scope, and do not always include formal assessment. As recently as 1975, one in three British medical schools offered no specified training in communication skills. Traditionally, doctors have developed such facility for communication as they possess by trial and error as they practised. Gradually, the need to acquire the necessary professional knowledge, skills, and attitudes—to learn the scientific basis from which the art of competent communication is derived—has been recognized.

This small book attempts to distil these elements into a concise form, as free from jargon as possible, to aid the student who seeks to develop skill as a communicator. While it is intended primarily to be of assistance to undergraduates, I hope it will interest practising doctors who are still alive to the need for continued learning.

BENEFITS FROM COMMUNICATION SKILLS

Before going further, it is worthwhile to look at the benefits that can accrue from acquiring interviewing skills. Good communication is not an esoteric theoretical objective, nor is it just about becoming a more understanding and approachable doctor (though that is a likely bonus). It is about being a more efficient doctor. Communication is, to put it simply, the key to effectiveness for the doctor as a professional.

First, communication skill is an absolute requirement in obtaining a good history from the patient. This information alone, if gathered and assessed with care, provides a correct diagnosis in more than a half of all patients [5], and in as many as four out of five general medical cases [6].

Second, communication skill constitutes one of the corner-stones of therapy. Most consultations end with what may be called the *exposition* [7], during which the doctor offers his assessment of the case and outlines proposed treatment. Rapport, confidence, and trust are necessary for the patient to respond to the doctor's advice, understand the nature of his illness, comply with specific recommendations made, take (and continue to take) any medication prescribed—as well as a clear grasp of the doctor's instructions. These elements in the relationship also have therapeutic value, and may contribute directly to the patient's recovery.

Commonly, too, a doctor's recommendations include educational advice aimed at modifying the patient's way of life—advice to change eating patterns, take more exercise or rest, avoid recourse to alcohol, curtail smoking, avoid certain forms of stress, and so on. This educational advice can be expected to have an impact only if the relationship between doctor and patient rests on mutual confidence and respect, and if the patient's attitude to his illness is known and understood by the doctor.

Good communication between doctor and patient indirectly affords a further important benefit, for the doctor at least: it makes it much less likely that dissatisfaction with the doctor's professional services will end in litigation. The experience of the medical protection societies has provided clear evidence that, although no doctor is immune from making a mistake, a lawsuit is much more likely when communication between doctor and patient, or between doctor and doctor, has been poor. Their experience also underlines the protective value of good written communication in the patient's records and in correspondence between doctors. The important function of the written record is discussed later.

Lastly, it is worth pointing out, as Enelow and Swisher have done [8], that doctors' claims to leadership of the health team—to a co-ordinating role among the other caring professionals—rest on their ability to function as the principal communicators. Unless that role is competently performed, the claim is a sham!

POOR COMMUNICATION

So much for the positive side of the coin. When the effects of poor communication are considered, it becomes even more clear that communication is at the heart of a sound doctor–patient relationship. As already indicated, when patients have the opportunity to criticize their doctors, their dissatisfactions usually centre not around the doctor's technical competence, but around his inadequacies as a communicator. The sorts of criticism that are expressed have been summarized in numerous published reports, including those of Cartwright [9], Dunkelmans [10], Hawkins [11], Parkin [12], and Reynolds [13]. They are concerned with doctors' unapproachability and with the inadequate explanations that patients often feel they are given regarding investigations undertaken when they are unwell and the nature of their illnesses [11,14].

'My doctor? Oh, he's thorough enough, but he's not the listening sort. I couldn't talk to *him* about *that*!'

'Of course, they looked after me superbly in hospital, but they never actually *tell* you *anything*. And you don't like to ask, do you?'

'He just gave me the prescription, and out I came. Nothing was said about what's *really* wrong with me. And I never got a chance to try to tell him how I was feeling.'

But in contemporary practice, more and more patients want to be involved in decisions about their own bodies, and to participate intelligently in their own care and treatment. This is an inevitable and wholly desirable consequence of improved education and greater health consciousness among the population. It is demonstrated by the popularity of health foods, health clubs, and activities such as jogging, not to mention the proliferation of alternative forms of medicine.

The deficiencies, then, identified by some patients relate particularly to the handling of the affective aspects of health and illness, to discussion of their close personal relationships, or of their emotional reactions to ill health: worry, grave anxiety, and the fear of disability, pain, loss of employment, or death, are some of the more serious concerns.

OBSTACLES TO COMMUNICATION

Two topics associated with the greatest reticence are death and sexuality, which are identified as 'problem' topics that are difficult to discuss with patients by both medical students [15] and junior doctors [16]. These are subjects which most human beings find it difficult to speak about openly and honestly, even with close friends. This aversion is greatly intensified when the prospect of death or sexual dysfunction has become a threat to the patient's well-being.

There are, of course, many medical interviews in which neither death and suffering nor sexuality enter the dialogue in any way whatsoever. But the inhibitions that surround these topics specifically are such that they can lead to a reluctance to become involved with *any* of the patient's feelings. In consequence, a greater distance is maintained in the professional relationship.

Besides, there are particular reasons why doctors find difficulty in talking about death and sexuality in a professional context. Later chapters consider in more detail the reasons why these topics are such sensitive areas, and consider ways in which such sources of 'discomfort' can be handled with greater ease and skill.

It can be argued that the apparent disparity between some doctors' technical competence on the one hand, and their skill in handling the affective aspects of illness on the other, is simply a reflection of the traditional dominance of the physical sciences in pre-clinical teaching, largely at the expense of applied behavioural science. The imbalance, a legacy of the educational 'model' advocated by Flexner [17], is slowly changing, but this is not the whole story. It will become evident that a number of other important factors can make the doctor ill at ease with patients' feelings, and therefore reluctant to discuss or take account of them.

2 Doctors' and patients' roles

To understand more clearly how doctors and patients interact, it is helpful to specify what is special about the doctor–patient relationship. Just as the pattern of communication affects a relationship, so the relationship, in a circular interaction, shapes and influences the manner of communication. How do the doctor and the patient, as they interact, view themselves and one another? In other words, what can be said about the doctor's professional role and the patient's sick role? Let us consider the patient first.

THE SICK ROLE

By speaking of the patient's role as that of a sick person, the intention is not to present a stereotyped view of how a patient does or should react to illness. On the contrary, the reader is likely to have recognized already that different individuals react in very different ways when they feel, or think they are, ill.

However, most people who are unwell look to the doctor for help, advice, or reassurance, and so they assume, as a sick person, a dependent role. This 'submission' to their medical attendant derives from the feelings of uncertainty and fear that come with illness. In turn, the patient's dependence tends to boost the doctor's self-assurance. Such words as 'I am in your hands, doctor. I'll just take your advice' do a great deal for the doctor's morale.

Occasionally, the patient is so anxious to be helpful to the doctor (and thereby to speed recovery) that he may be reluctant to deny having *any* symptom that is mentioned to him during questioning, and thus may seriously mislead the doctor. For this reason, 'leading' questions that invite a particular answer should be avoided, especially when the patient is initially describing his complaints.

Sometimes, patients are only too ready to adopt the sick role as a means of escape from the pressures of life, at home or at work.

Others find being 'unwell' the only sure way of gaining the attention and concern of those around them; these attention-seekers may enjoy recurrent ill health for year after year!

Among the more strange historical examples of sickness behaviour is the story of Florence Nightingale, who, after displaying immense courage, determination, and capability during her nursing career, took to her bed and remained there for a considerable part of her life, although still in good physical health. Another bizarre pattern is seen in the so-called Munchausen syndrome [18]. Occasional individuals are encountered in various fields of practice who repeatedly, and often very cunningly, secure their admission to hospital by falsifying the signs and symptoms of serious disease in themselves or, even more strangely, in their children [19].

In contrast, a few patients find difficulty in acknowledging that they are ill, and resist the sick role. Some of them are playing the ostrich, and refusing to face the possibility of disability or death. Some are acting bravely to try to protect their spouse or other loved ones from being upset by possible bad news. It is noteworthy that those whose everyday work centres on physical fitness, such as physiotherapists, athletes, physical instructors, and professional soldiers, often find the greatest difficulty in coming to terms with the idea that they are unwell. They regard health with such positive value that they are reluctant to acknowledge the fact of being ill.

THE DOCTOR'S 'PROFESSIONAL' ROLE

The notion of being a professional has several different dimensions. It signifies an area of competence, within which the professional has both responsibility and authority, and so a doctor is expected to take charge of the interview with his patient and to be capable of helping him. It also signifies a degree of controlled concern for the client (patient) but at the same time a formality, an unemotional correctness of manner, and a degree of detachment. To call a relationship 'professional' is to imply that it lacks the open feeling and warmth of a normal human relationship. Hence, the SAS man, after taking out a few terrorists in an eruption of ruthless violence, is spoken of as 'doing a professional job'.

Now if the term 'professional' can convey these overtones of detachment, the world 'clinical' has also, in general parlance, come to imply even more strongly a cool, almost indifferent competence. Thus, when a few years ago a prisoner was executed in Florida in the electric chair in the presence of public representatives, their leader was happy to emerge afterwards and reassure waiting reporters that it had all been carried out 'clinically'! That episode illustrated vividly the ordinary person's appreciation of the clinical atmosphere that doctors can unwittingly create—efficient certainly, but aloof and depersonalized.

Why, then, do these unfeeling attributes come to be associated with doctors' day-to-day working style, so providing some grounds for the criticisms, referred to in Chapter 1, that patients make of medical practitioners? It could be argued that, even from the patients' point of view, a degree of controlled clinical detachment is necessary to create the freedom for patients to share their problems with a doctor, knowing that he is not expected to shoulder the whole burden of their distress. It is essential to understand more clearly the nature of the balance between detachment and involvement if doctors are to become better communicators, and if the divergence between patients' needs and expectations and doctors' apparent performance is to be reconciled. To do this, it is helpful to look at the factors that significantly influence doctors' professional behaviour, and that therefore shape their clinical style and determine their ability to become involved with the affective aspects of illness.

FACTORS INHIBITING COMMUNICATION

There are several factors that, consciously or unconsciously, may inhibit affective communication between doctor and patient. The first and simplest is *time*, or the lack of it. For most doctors, time is a precious commodity which has to be rationed out over the commitments of the day, while some is kept in reserve for the unexpected 'extra'. This pressure of time inevitably creates a reluctance on the part of the doctor to become involved in peripheral matters, inessentials, or irrelevancies. The patient's personal concerns may (unfortunately) be seen as falling into these categories.

Patients are likely to be inhibited from expressing their worries and other feelings by the sense that the doctor is short of time. If there are other patients sitting in the waiting room, it may seem selfish to take up what they feel is a disproportionate share of the doctor's time.

'You're always such a busy person, doctor. I don't want to take up more of your time today.'

'I'm sure you've got more important things to attend to than my little worries.'

As well as this practical problem of pressure of time, two other factors, already mentioned, can inhibit affective communication between doctor and patient because of the uncomfortable, and at times intolerable, feelings that they are able to endanger within the professional relationship. These are suffering and death on one hand, and sexuality on the other.

Death and suffering

All doctors need some protective insulation from the distressing feelings that pain, suffering, and death inevitably give rise to during the course of serious illness. These emotions are especially difficult for doctors to live with because they are likely to feel that it is their professional responsibility to prevent suffering, and that death in particular is the ultimate failure in medical practice.

But whatever the doctor's attitudes towards death and suffering, he cannot be expected to carry the burden of the distress created by illness, and may have learnt to protect himself from these painful feelings by avoiding involvement in the affective aspects of his patients' ill health. In consequence, he has distanced himself from the patient as a person, so that he can feel less closely involved. Maguire [20] described how both doctors and nurses usually distance themselves from patients who are terminally ill, to ensure their own emotional survival.

Sexuality

A second source of professionally unacceptable or intolerable feelings is sexuality. Clinical practice regularly exposes doctors to degrees of nudity and intimate forms of touching that in any other private setting would be permitted only to a lover and would be associated with sexual arousal (Fig. 2.1). This intimacy of clinical

Fig. 2.1 Coping with the intimacy of clinical examination

practice has to be professionalized to render it secure and emotion-
ally comfortable for both doctor and patient. How this is achieved
is not taught explicitly, but is usually learnt by example. A great
deal of the impersonal formality of doctors' professional style
relates to the need to desexualize the closeness of clinical contact
(see page 63).

In various ways, then, doctors contrive to become indifferent to
nudity and intimate touching in a professional setting. However,
they may achieve this professionalism only through an unwillingness
to think about the patient as a sexual person, thereby excluding the
patient's sexuality from consideration or discussion. At the worst,
these influences mean that the doctor eliminates all warmth from
his professional manner, and in some instances make open discussion of sexual problems unthinkable for him.

An understanding of the part these factors play in inhibiting
affective communication is so important that I shall return to them
at a later stage.

THE WARD ENVIRONMENT

Those who are starting to work in hospital may not at first recognize that the ward environment itself should be included among the potential obstacles to good communication between patient and doctor. When patients are admitted to a ward, they sense that they have, willy-nilly, become part of a close-knit group. They quickly begin to recognize the daily routines of life in the ward, to which they are expected to conform. They cannot fail to become aware of other patients, some of whom may be more ill than themselves. At the same time, they can readily see how busy the medical and nursing staff are.

In such an environment, patients almost inevitably feel under pressure not to be too demanding, not to take up too much of the staff's time, to contain their worries, and certainly to express them only to the 'correct' person at the proper time. Both patients and staff tend to have an image of the 'good' patient—helpful, pleasant, and, as far as possible, uncomplaining, if not downright stoical! Thus, one can often hear phrases such as: 'I hope I'll be a good patient, nurse.' 'Can you *spare* just a minute, doctor?' 'If it's not too much *trouble*.' 'I hope I'm not making a *fuss*'.

At the same time, the hospital environment is likely to intensify the patient's emotional vulnerability. There is a loss of independence, and even identity, which is made worse by shedding one's normal clothes and facing the world in night-clothes, which may themselves belong to the hospital. Each patient has to try to work out who is who in the hierarchy of the ward. It is akin to the feeling that most medical students feel on the first day *they* find themselves in a ward, uncertain of who the staff are and of the rules of the organization. In such a situation, every aspect of the environment begins to assume great importance and every communication is liable to be distorted by anxiety or the desire to conform.

The ward round

The main contact the patient has with the medical staff is usually during ward rounds. The patient is confronted with a group of people, rather than an individual. There is less privacy, and little intimacy. The encounter is likely to have an aura of protocol, rank, and formality. Often the inter- and intra-professional communication between doctor and nurse, and between consultant, registrar, house-officer, and student, takes precedence over unhurried sensitive communication with the patient. The group on the round is liable to cluster together near the foot of the bed, and the centre of interest may be more the case record, and the latest investigative reports, than the anxious and hesitant individual in the bed.

If, during a ward round the patient indicates a desire to talk, it is important that the senior person present should sit down close to the head of the bed and try to meet the need for unhurried 'private' conversation. Sometimes it is impossible to achieve the appropriate degree of privacy and intimacy in an open ward; it is best then to talk with the patient again after the ward round is completed, in the privacy of a side room or office.

3 Conducting an interview

Before considering the conduct of an interview in detail, it is useful to look at the elements involved in interpersonal communication. They include both verbal and non-verbal 'messages', which may be classified into four varieties.

(1) *verbal*: the choice of spoken words;

(2) *intonational*: the pitch, tone, or cadence of speech, the modulation of the voice; the whisper of confidentiality; the rising crescendo of anger or concern; the flat tones of despair;

(3) *paralinguistic*: non-verbal sound or utterances, e.g. the noncommittal nasal 'hm-hm'; the sharp inspiration of surprise—'phew'; the expiratory puff signifying disgust;

(4) *kinesic*: communication through movements, facial expressions, posture or gesture—'body language'. (An excellent popular account of this aspect of communication may be found in Desmond Morris's *Manwatching* [21].)

While all these elements play a part in medical interviews, the learner should pay particular attention to body language, the unspoken messages conveyed without sound. In particular, he should be alert to any incongruity between what the patient is saying aloud and what his body is actually 'saying'. Tense knuckles, a furrowed brow, folded arms, or foot tapping, for example, may be conveying a message quite different from the patient's words. The student should never forget that his own body language is, in turn, communicating messages to the patient that may facilitate or inhibit communication between them.

Some specific points about body language are emphasized in the next section, which considers in detail the conduct of an interview.

THE PHYSICAL SETTING

Communication can be helped or hindered by the physical setting in which the interview is being conducted. Normally, patient and doctor should be comfortably seated at the same level (Fig. 3.1). A possible exception to this arrangement might occur when the patient is sitting *higher* than the doctor, for example on the edge of the couch after physical examination has been completed. If in bed, the patient should be encouraged to sit up wherever possible and made comfortable with pillow support, while the doctor draws up a chair alongside the bed.

Fig. 3.1   Appropriate seating for good communication

The two chairs should usually be arranged four to five feet apart, and set at an angle to each other, so that a direct face-to-face confrontation is avoided, but without a desk or other major piece of furniture intervening. In this position, the doctor and patient can easily make and break eye-to-eye contact, without any awkwardness. Exceptionally, it may be appropriate for the doctor to position his chair directly in front of a patient, for instance if he is speaking to a very old person whose body movements are restricted, whose hearing is poor, or whose attention is impaired because of senile confusion or dementia.

The sort of interview arrangement that can have the most deleterious effects on communication is that in which the doctor faces the patient from behind a large desk piled with desk calendars, reference books, or even a vase of flowers, and beyond which the patient perches on a small plain chair, like a pupil in a headteacher's study.

Fig. 3.2 The headmasterly 'I am in charge' setting: a grave barrier to communication

Ideally, no one else should be present. If a nurse is in the room, she should have been clearly briefed to follow the conversation discreetly, and to leave the room if sensitive personal topics are raised or if the patient shows any hesitation in speaking to the doctor. A student or trainee, if present, should be introduced by name, and should sit near the doctor, but a little farther from the patient, within the same arc that the patient's chair is facing. From this position, the student can easily exchange eye-to-eye contact with patient and so participate in the interview, whether joining in the dialogue or not.

THE INTRODUCTION

At the outset, doctor and patient may sometimes be old acquaintances, but will often be complete strangers. When they are acquainted, their familiarity with each other socially may be an obstacle to an effective therapeutic relationship, since a less clinical atmosphere obtains.

The doctor should observe the patient closely as he enters the room. The patient's gait and posture, style of dress, manner, and facial expressions can provide important clues about the reason for the consultation. While these points are being noted, the patient is guided to a chair. If the doctor has never met the patient before, the introductory exchange should centre around 'Who are you?' before the presenting complaint ('How are you?') is discussed.

In a hospital clinic, a helpful introduction may be to say something like 'Good morning, Mr Smith. I am Dr Brown. I see you've brought a letter from Dr Green. Let me see what she has to tell me.' This allows the doctor a few moments to read through the letter of referral, while at the same time continuing to observe the patient's demeanour. Then enquiries about the patient's occupation, age, marital status (and, if married, 'Have you a family?') should be made. This initial exploration of 'Who are you?', suitably phrased in a friendly, open way, helps to put the patient at ease, provides the doctor with valuable background information, but also indicates to the patient from the outset that the doctor is concerned with him or her as a *person*, and is ready to talk about wider aspects of the patient's situation, not just the immediate complaint.

THE CORE OF THE INTERVIEW

After the introductory phase of the interview, the questions to be explored first can be phrased as:

(1) 'What is your problem?'

(2) 'How has it affected you?'

'*What is your problem*?' This question can be expressed in a number of ways, and the word 'problem' need not be used. 'What brings you to see me?' 'What can I do to help you?' 'What do you feel is wrong with yourself?' These are examples of how an open question can invite the patient to express what the trouble is. It is best to put aside one's pen as the question is asked.

Sometimes the patient has more than one problem and, while each should be noted, it may be necessary in the time available to concentrate on the immediate problem, or the main problem, and to plan a later interview to investigate other concerns the patient has mentioned.

One must be mindful, too, that the problem with which the patient presents may not in fact be the patient's real underlying problem. The patient may be using the presenting problem as a visiting card, a safe way of establishing contact to find out what sort of person the doctor is—how approachable, how understanding. Only then will the patient decide whether to reveal what the *real* problem is. For example, the teenager complaining of a mild vaginal discharge may in fact be anxious to discover whether she is pregnant, or whether she dare ask the doctor for contraceptive advice. The middle-aged man ostensibly complaining of tiredness or insomnia may be trying to pluck up courage to speak to the doctor about his erectile impotence. The patient with vague breathlessness may be too afraid to mention directly the lump she has felt in her breast.

For each complaint or problem, more detailed information should be sought, as Maguire and Rutter have described [22]. Accurate information, as far as this is possible, about the time of onset and the timing of subsequent developments and effects is usually of considerable diagnostic value. These details are set out more fully in the Appendix.

As well as obtaining an objective account of the sequence of events, it is often worthwhile eliciting the patient's subjective interpretation of the onset of the illness or problem: 'Did anything seem to start it off?', 'What seemed to start it off?', or (particularly if the disorder is not apparently due to organic disease) 'What do *you* think started it off?' Giving the patient the opportunity to express his views on the cause and nature of his indisposition can be valuable in preventing mistakes or misunderstandings, and often throws light on the diagnosis. The verbal expressions and imagery used by a patient to describe symptoms can reveal something about how the illness is perceived and the degree of anxiety it has generated: 'The pain keeps gnawing away, as if it was eating into my bones.' 'I get these electric shock feelings in my head, and the top of my head prickles all over.' 'When the pain comes on, I feel absolutely lifeless. My whole body begins to go cold from the waist downwards.'

When a complaint is of longer standing, or when the patient has apparently come to consult the doctor out of the blue, it is often revealing to enquire 'What made you decide to do something about it *now*?'

'*How has this affected you*?' An open question of this sort, introduced relatively early in the interview, is designed specifically to invite the patient to express his emotional response to the illness. Sometimes, an open question initially produces a non-committal response or a denial of affect from the patient. If so, a secondary and more specific enquiry later in the interview may help the patient respond, for example 'And how have you been feeling in yourself?' or 'How have you been able to cope?' or, more directly and empathically, 'You must have felt quite alarmed?'; or even, in certain situations, something like 'You must have been feeling at the end of your tether?'

'SYSTEMATIC' INTERVIEWING

At this stage in the history, having heard the patient's account of the presenting complaint or problem, the student or inexperienced doctor tends to follow a predetermined outline for the rest of the interview. This is generally based on a sequence of headings, covering the full content of a comprehensive history, i.e. a review of the function of the main organ systems; past medical history; family history; social history. Because he has been taught what a complete medical history should comprise, a learner may be at pains to ensure that every area is covered and that no detail of possible importance is omitted (see Appendix).

By following a structured pattern through the interview, the student is given a greater sense of confidence. Most students are anxious when they first embark upon solo interviews with patients. They may be afraid that they could lose control of the interview, or forget what to ask next and therefore 'dry up'. In the back of their minds is a fairly long checklist of questions, which they tend to work steadily through.

This approach, which can easily become a habit, results in a structured interrogation of the patient, who is expected to answer a long succession of direct, closed questions. These may appear to the patient to have little or no relevance to his immediate concerns and complaints. If the interviewer adopts an interrogatory style from the very beginning, tightly controlling the sequence of question and answer, anxious not to lose the thread as he ploughs through his checklist of topics, the patient is unlikely to have adequate opportunity to express his problems. The style of the interview will stifle expression of the affective aspects of the patient's illness.

If direct questioning of a systematic nature has to be included in a consultation, the guiding principle is that such questions should be tagged on to the latter part of the interview, after the patient has been given the chance to respond to more open questions in his own words.

---

1. Comprehensive systematic history-taking

   then

2. Systematic clinical examination

   then

3. A wide range of potentially relevant investigations

   then

4. Diagnostic reasoning based on all the above information

Fig. 3.3 Model of the 'systematic' approach to diagnosis

ALTERNATIVE MODELS OF DIAGNOSTIC REASONING

The systematic, comprehensive method of history-taking and clinical examination referred to above is taught traditionally to students as part of their initiation into clinical work. Every student, of course, needs to become familiar with the language of all aspects of history-taking, and with a great variety of normal as well as abnormal physical findings. For this purpose, unselective overall enquiries and examination provide excellent basic practice.

However, this approach to diagnosis is certainly not adopted during consultation by experienced clinicians. If only to avoid wasting time, the blunderbuss approach with a full detailed history, top-to-toe clinical examination, and a battery of all potentially relevant investigations has to be replaced by more economical methods. Furthermore, experience brings an awareness that diagnosis is not an end in itself (apart from the intellectual self-satisfaction it affords). Diagnosis is, in effect, a statement of probability which forms the basis on which decisions about management are made. In these practical terms, a satisfactory diagnosis does not have to be absolutely certain. However, the assumed diagnosis must ensure that the patient will be better managed on the basis of that assumption rather than on any alternative conclusion. Macartney [23] emphasized and illustrated this point very clearly.

Review of the pattern of working of more skilled and experienced doctors has allowed their methods of history-taking and diagnostic reasoning to be analysed in some detail [24,25,26]. The patterns revealed are quite different from the systematic model described above and illustrated schematically in Fig. 3.3. Various attempts have been made to outline the stages and steps involved in diagnostic reasoning. Of the different 'models' of diagnostic logic, the following are now well recognized.

Diagnostic algorithms

The notion underlying a diagnostic algorithm is in essence the flow-chart adopted in certain types of digital computer programs. With its aid, a decision-tree can be created, leading by alternative pathways towards different diagnoses. Figures 3.4 and 3.5 are examples of diagnostic algorithms published in the *British Medical Journal*.

This analytical model allows an economy of reasoning and a precision of diagnosis that is very attractive but that is just not possible in many cases. However, algorithms can sometimes provide clear guidelines for dealing with particular clinical problems, and so help the learner to adopt the skills of the expert.

The hypothetico-deductive model

Clinicians who view medicine as Science are pleased to invest their diagnostic reasoning with a scientific aura. According to this model, the diagnostic process begins by collecting observations about the patient (from the history and initial examination). From these observations, the clinician generates a number of diagnostic hypotheses (usually not more than four or five) to explain the observations made. These hypotheses can spring from the doctor's experience, hunch, or even intuition [27,28]. He then seeks to eliminate or confirm the various possibilities by further observations, tests, and investigations. In this model, the generation and testing of hypotheses is seen as the scientific 'core' of diagnostic reasoning (Fig. 3.6).

The probabilistic model (Bayes' theorem)

The theorem of Bayes (which few clinicians have heard of, and even fewer understand!) calculates the probability of a future event on the basis of prior probabilities of associated past events. In the diagnostic context, Bayesian analysis allows the probabilities of different diagnoses in a particular patient to be calculated (and therefore ranked) from the known features of the clinical presentation of other patients previously evaluated. The validity of this model has been clearly demonstrated by its successful application in computer programs for the elucidation of everyday diagnostic problems such as the diagnosis of abdominal pain [29,30] and of congenital heart disease [31].

The basic requirement for precise application of Bayes' theorem is a bank of data that can be represented as a conditional probability matrix, of which Fig. 3.7 is a notional example relating to some of the features present in a population of patients complaining of vaginal discharge. From such a tabulation, using Bayes' theorem, the probability of each diagnosis can be calculated for an individual patient with a particular combination of symptoms.

In day-to-day practice, clinicians do not, of course, engage in mathematical computation in this precise way, but sometimes the pattern of their diagnostic reasoning follows a Bayesian model. They have accumulated from past experience a mental databank of

Fig. 3.4 Example of a diagnostic algorithm, outlining the diagnosis of vaginal discharge. (Reproduced from the *British Medical Journal* by kind permission)

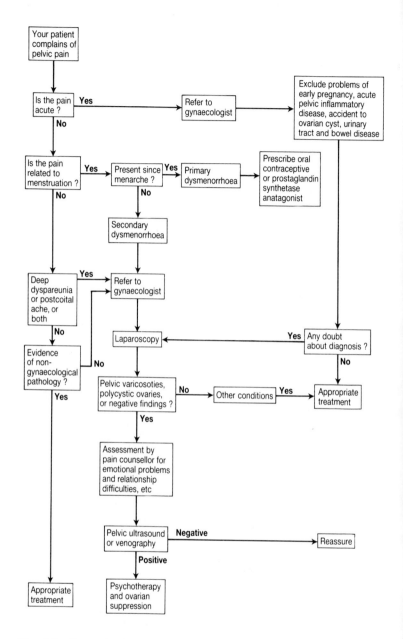

Fig. 3.5 Example of a diagnostic algorithm, outlining the diagnosis of pelvic pain. (Reproduced from the *British Medical Journal* by kind permission)

1. Eliciting the presenting complaints

   then

2. Forming a number of diagnostic hypotheses

   then

3. Seeking to validate or negate these hypotheses by
   selective questioning
   selective physical examination
   selective investigations

Fig. 3.6 Model of the hypothetico-deductive approach to diagnosis.

	Trichomonas	Thrush	Anaerobic vaginitis	Gonorrhoea	Chlamydia
Yellow discharge	74	12	42	27	24
Itching	86	95	2	2	4
Odour	94	3	97	4	5
Dyspareunia	62	88	5	6	7

Fig. 3.7 Percentage frequency (notional) of certain symptoms associated with various causes of vaginal discharge

1. Eliciting the presenting complaints

   then

2. Forming a short list of probable diagnoses, based
   on the doctor's knowledge of clinical epidemiology

   then

3. Eliciting futher clinical information selectively, to
   refine the estimate of diagnostic probabilities

Fig. 3.8 Model of the probabilistic (Bayesian) approach to diagnosis impressions, correlating certain clinical findings with particular diagnoses. They selectively elicit information about those parameters they have found to have the greatest discriminatory power. In this way, they mentally juggle with a league-table of probable diagnoses [23] (Fig. 3.8). Using the same example as in Fig. 3.7, if a patient complains of vaginal discharge, the doctor will have several possibilities in mind. The discharge is described as yellow: thrush infection seems a low probability. Is dyspareunia (painful intercourse) present? No: thrush infection is therefore doubly unlikely. Is the discharge malodourous? Yes: trichomonal infection or anaerobic infection are now emerging as the most probable diagnoses. Is there itching? No: anaerobic vaginitis thus emerges as the most likely cause of the patient's symptoms on the basis of the selective enquiries made. Confirmatory tests (microscopy for 'clue' cells, amine test) could put the matter beyond reasonable doubt.

DOVE-TAILING THE HISTORY TAKING AND CLINICAL EXAMINATION

In practice, the history taking and clinical examination are generally not separate consecutive parts of the consultation; they proceed alongside each other as complementary parts of the process of diagnostic reasoning.

The degree of overlap between history taking and examination is considerably influenced by the nature and site of the patient's complaint. If, for example, the patient complains of a sore eye, or a painful toe, or a skin eruption on the hands, the doctor will want to begin examining the affected part early in the consultation. If, on the other hand, it is clear from the nature of the presenting symptoms that the patient will have to undress completely for a more comprehensive examination, the doctor will probably prefer to proceed as far as possible with his diagnostic questioning before asking the patient to undress.

Even if the doctor feels he has completed the formal history-taking before he embarks on the physical examination, he should nevertheless continue to communicate sensitively during the examination itself. If either patient or doctor feels awkward with the intimacy attending undressing and physical examination, this is likely to create an obstacle to continuing communication. Initially, then, the patient should be told clearly how much undressing is necessary—what to take off, and perhaps what to leave on. 'I'd like you to take off everything except your underpants.' 'Please take off your shoes, tights and pants so that I can examine you.'

In this situation, the learner has to avoid adopting an exaggerated and distant formality, in which the silence is broken only by an occasional curt instruction: 'Take a deep breath.' 'Again.' However, attempts to overcome awkwardness with a stream of distracting social chit-chat about irrelevant topics such as the weather, or holidays, are not helpful. To avoid a silence, which would be both embarrassing and probably alarming, the patient could be asked, for example, more detailed questions about his job, or a parent could be asked about his or her children. If through professional skill a comfortable sense of relaxed intimacy is created during the physical examination, the patient will be more willing to voice worrying or delicate concerns.

It is helpful to explain to the patient what you are about to do *before* you do it, and this is especially important if the patient cannot easily see what is happening. This applies, for instance, when firm palpation or percussion over the spine is to be performed, or when, with the patient in the left lateral position, rectal examination is to be undertaken. Particularly during physical examination, the doctor should choose simple words and phrases that the patient can easily understand and that will not cause alarm or embarrassment. During clinical examination, the patient's anxiety about what the doctor is perhaps going to discover can be quite intense, and questions can readily acquire a threatening implication. For example, a patient may be caused alarm if she were asked during auscultation of the heart whether there was a family history of heart disease, or if, during vaginal examination, she was suddenly asked 'Have you ever had a cervical smear?' In each instance, the patient might well jump to the conclusion that the doctor had found something ominous.

SELECTIVE BUT SENSITIVE ENQUIRIES

At the beginning of the interview the initiative is with the patient and the doctor is mainly an observant listener, but during the second phase of the consultation the initiative moves to the doctor, who has to direct his questions selectively as the process of diagnosis advances.

But although the doctor is very much in the driving seat during the heart of the consultation, the open and sensitive approach taken during the initial unfolding of the presenting problem is still required. The manner and content of the patient's responses to these selective questions may provide an indication of the patient's feelings, which the doctor should be alert to recognize, responding appropriately. The degree of openness with which questions are posed can help or hinder the expression of feeling. For example, it is often helpful to ask 'Have you always enjoyed good health?' rather than 'What previous illnesses or operations have you had?' Answers to the first question are more likely to reveal something of patients' attitudes towards their general health. Similarly, it is better to ask 'Do the members of your family all enjoy good health?' rather than asking only about particular diseases.

THE VALUE OF EXPERIENCE

The application of all forms of diagnostic reasoning in a selective but reliable way depends crucially upon a good knowledge of the natural history of disease, and especially of the manner in which it presents. Such knowledge is an essential element in all the diagnostic models reviewed above. It may be structured as an algorithm; it may involve pattern recognition—the significance of particular clusters of clinical features; or it may provide the basis of a statistical assessment of probabilities in the circumstances of a particular case. As the student's knowledge of medicine grows and the diagnostic logic at his disposal is refined, redundant steps in the diagnostic process can be avoided. The whole procedure of consultation becomes quicker, more efficient, and more cost-effective as superfluous diagnostic enquiries and investigations are eliminated.

However, diagnosis cannot always be reached by the sort of elegant definitive analysis provided by some of the above models. Students should not be discouraged if sometimes they have just to gather *all* the information they can about the patient and then plan a relatively wide range of investigations.

With increasing experience, a doctor comes to understand not only the natural history of disease but also the way in which people tend to react to health problems. He begins to recognize that patients react both to their own illnesses and also to those of other family members, friends, and neighbours. For example, the death of a parent or close sibling during childhood often leaves a legacy of insecurity or depression; the fact that her mother had a hysterectomy may leave a patient with a niggling apprehension that the same thing will happen to her; breast cancer in a friend or neighbour may trigger off the anxiety underlying a patient's present complaints.

CONCLUDING THE INTERVIEW

Before the consultation ends, it is often worth while to pose a further open question such as 'Well, have we covered all aspects of the problem?' or 'Have you anything more you want to tell me?' This helps to ensure that patients who have been slow to respond earlier in the interview, or who may have forgotten something regarded as important, have another opportunity to state what is on their mind. It can be particularly important when interviewing an anxious or elderly, forgetful person.

So far, we have attempted to set out some sort of plan for a medical interview, intended to facilitate good communication between patient and doctor and in particular to provide clear opportunities for the patient to speak about attitudes and feelings surrounding the illness. The following basic elements have been identified.

- A comfortable supportive physical setting.
- A warm introduction, to elicit a response to 'Who are you?'
- An open initial enquiry, allowing the patient every opportunity to present the problem in his own words.
- A specific invitation to describe any affective responses to illness.
- A sequence of selective questions in the search for a diagnosis, usually supplemented by initial clinical examination.
- If there is time, in the latter part of the interview, some systematic questioning to complete a comprehensive overview of the patient.
- Concluding 'open' questions.

This model is incomplete in one important respect. No individual interview, with its exploration of a particular patient's problem(s), can be expected always to follow a predetermined pattern. Unexpected information may begin to emerge, and the patient may react in an unexpected way to certain questions, providing verbal or non-verbal clues.

No model of a good medical interview, therefore, can be tied in a rigid way to a completely pre-arranged structure. An essential feature is the responsiveness of the doctor (see p. 50), and his awareness that at any point the patient might reveal a clue, or drop a cue that the doctor must be ready to recognize and respond to, branching away from the planned pattern of the interview to follow a different line of enquiry. Such responsiveness is discussed in more detail in Chapter 6.

4 Facilitating communication

After reviewing the broad strategy of the interview, we need to look at the tactics of the dialogue. Of particular importance are the methods by which a doctor can facilitate communication and so elicit as accurately as possible in the time available the information needed to make a diagnosis and plan treatment, while giving the patient adequate opportunity to express his feelings. Whatever the nature of the verbal exchanges, the patient's body language, which may convey information of its own, must be continuously observed throughout.

VOCABULARY

The doctor should ask questions in clear, unambiguous language suitable to the patient's age, education, and cultural background; the information gained during the introductory phase of the interview about the patient's general background will be of assistance. The vocabulary chosen should not include technical terms or unfamiliar words. If the doctor senses that the patient is hesitating for want of suitable vocabulary, he should attempt to include the needed non-technical words in his questions. This applies especially to enquiries about sexual function. When the doctor supplies in a comfortable, open way suitable simple but explicit words describing sexual function, this does more to facilitate discussion than merely providing a vocabulary.

The patient can follow the purpose and direction of the doctor's enquiries more readily if the pattern of questions follows some logical grouping and sequence. If the doctor does have an afterthought, he should explain himself; he might say 'Now could we just go back to this question of your indigestion? Was there ever a time when food actually seemed to stick in your throat?'

Topics that the patient may feel sensitive about should usually be introduced in the latter part of an interview, when confidence and rapport have been established. Again, they should wherever possible form part of a logical sequence of related enquiries. For example, questions about urinary or faecal incontinence should follow enquiries about normal excretory function, and questions about dyspareunia (painful intercourse) can follow those about other types of pelvic pain, pruritus vulvae, or similar pelvic complaints.

Not all patients are reluctant to speak frankly and freely to a doctor. Some may be so ready to talk that the doctor's problem is to control their garrulous chatter. However, much greater skill is required to help a hesitant patient open up.

CAUSES OF RETICENCE

It is first all-important to try to recognize *why* a patient is holding back or having difficulty in expressing himself freely, so that whenever possible something can be done about the inhibiting factor(s). The patient's reticence may be due to the following.

- The presence of a third party: a nurse, a student, or even an accompanying relative. They should, if necessary, be asked to leave the room.
- Sometimes the fact that the doctor is also the family doctor may inhibit an adolescent from speaking freely.
- The patient may fear that revealing his complaints will lead to the realization of his worst fears: a diagnosis of serious disease, admission to hospital, an operation.
- A reluctance to take up the doctor's time with concerns that the patient may feel are undeserving of his time and attention: 'You are always a very busy man, doctor, and there are several folk still waiting to see you.'
- Embarrassment or shame about the nature of the complaint. This might apply to a wide range of disorders, but especially to those with a sexual association: venereal disease; other genital complaints; drinking problems; pregnancy in the unmarried, widowed, or separated; impotence.
- Cultural barriers. For example, many Asian women find it dif-

ficult to discuss personal or marital problems with a male doctor or even with a strange female doctor. A youthful or a venerable-looking doctor may be seen as an unsuitable confidant if he or she obviously belongs to a different generation from the patient.

These are some of the more specific obstacles to open communication that should be kept in mind if a patient is holding back. With experience and training, the student will learn to recognize the causes of reticence and be able to overcome them. The communication skills to be employed include non-verbal (body) language, speech, and appropriate use of silences.

WAYS OF FACILITATING COMMUNICATION

Non-verbal

An unhurried manner is a basic essential, conveying the message 'I have time to talk'. While listening, the doctor can nod attentively (but not nod off!). He should not be afraid to smile, since smiling is often the best way of conveying reassurance, understanding, and warmth. If the patient pauses, the doctor may lower his eyes for a moment without looking away and then look back at the patient's face, signalling 'Go on'. At certain points, it is helpful to discard pen and notes in an obvious way, and push them to one side, perhaps adding 'So tell me more about . . .', referring to a more sensitive topic that has not yet been ventilated adequately, and about which the doctor feels there is more to be said. If what seems a delicate question has to be posed, it can help to lean forward towards the patient, underlining the intimacy and confidentiality of the conversation.

By speech

A variety of simple short responses from the doctor will encourage the patient to continue speaking, especially if accompanied by a brief smile: 'Yes, I see', 'Go on', 'I understand', or sometimes 'I don't quite follow you', inviting the patient to give a fuller account.

Reflecting

Somewhat similarly, but more positively, the doctor can encourage the patient to continue speaking by repeating, and so *reflecting* back to him, a phrase, idea, or significant word from what the patient has just said. By picking up a word or expression in this way, the patient is prompted to express himself further.

Here is an example of this technique of reflecting.

'Doctor, I can always sense when my husband is building up towards another bout of heavy drinking, but . . . well . . . I just feel there's absolutely *nothing* I can do about it. I've given up.'
'Nothing?'
'Well . . . maybe. . . . You see, I'm always afraid if I say anything that I'll be to blame for what he's doing. Do you think I should try to talk to him?'

Another example might be the following interchange.

'The period pains are not too bad, but the headaches I get before the period starts to make me *desperately* miserable for three or four days every month.'
'You feel desperate at that time?'
'Yes, to be honest, I do. Recently there have been several times when I've thought of doing away with myself, because at the time it felt as if there was nothing to live for.'

Clarifying

This term is used to describe another ploy which helps to clarify to the patient what he is trying to put into words, and also allows the doctor to check on his own tentative deductions:

'You seem to be saying that, since the pains began, you not only gradually lost your appetite, but also lost interest in all kinds of everyday activities. Is that correct?'

Or, to offer another example:

'Are you trying to tell me that you're really afraid this is something very serious? Is that what you feel?'

Summarizing

It can also be very helpful, particularly when the history is long and complicated, to attempt at some point to summarize all or part of the patient's account of things. This recapitulation must be done tentatively, getting the patient to corroborate the more important details. Otherwise there is the danger that a compliant patient may just accept the doctor's version of the history, which could reflect more the doctor's preconceived ideas than what actually happened:

'So if we could just go over the main points of what you have told me so far. Your periods were perfectly normal and regular until five months ago. Then you missed two periods completely, and then bled heavily for three weeks. Since that time there has been some scanty loss most days, but no pain at any time. Is that correct?'

By appropriate use of silences

One of the nightmarish anxieties of the inexperienced student or doctor is that he will dry up during the interview; that he will run out of questions; and that an embarrassing silence will open up, creating discomfort and disrupting communication. In contrast, an easy interview often seems to flow along in sustained dialogue with barely a pause. The learner can avoid an undesirable hiatus of his own making by having in reserve one or two fill-in questions that cannot be answered very briefly (e.g. a question about the patient's childhood or about other family members) but which has some loose relevance to the presenting symptoms. One of these questions can be thrown in when such a silence threatens; while the patient is answering, the questioner can pick up the threads and poise himself for his next line of enquiry.

It is a mistake to believe that silences must be avoided at all costs. Apart from the nervous silences of the beginner referred to above, other silences can occur, when the patient runs out of words or is unsure about expressing his feelings. In this situation, the doctor must resist the temptation to disarm the silence promptly with a new question on a new topic, and so thereby suppress what the patient may be struggling to say. Rather, he should deliberately let the silence remain unbroken for a little time, while continuing to look at the patient with a facial expression of unhurried interest and concern.

FACILITATING THE OPEN EXPRESSION OF DEEP FEELINGS; MIRRORING AND CONFRONTATION

An interview in which the patient 'gets upset' is generally regarded as undesirable. Indeed, the very idea that the patient might burst into tears or erupt in anger would provide many inexperienced doctors with feelings of discomfort and embarrassment, or a sense of failure.

The same inhibitions about expressing emotions in the course of a formal professional consultation affect patients no less than doctors—'I'm sorry I got upset just now.' 'I shouldn't have let myself go like that—I feel ashamed.' 'I didn't want my feelings to get the better of me. I'd promised myself I wouldn't let that happen.' So, even when patients are experiencing strong feelings that are flooding up below the surface, they are likely to make every effort to restrain or conceal them, whereas the expression of the distressing feelings—the catharsis—may be an important part of the therapeutic value of the interview.

Hence, if the patient shows evidence of suppressed emotion, for example if tears begin to well up, the doctor must resist the temptation to jump in with distracting questions on a less emotive topic. He most certainly should not exhort such patients to cheer up, or to 'take a grip of themselves'.

As a first response to evidence of emotion, it is best if the doctor remains silent for a moment to allow the patient to stay with the feelings; to 'bridge' the silence the doctor should continue to look towards the patient with an expression of concern.

Mirroring

The patient is usually helped to put his feelings into words if the doctor acts as a sort of mirror in which the patient's feelings are revealed. The doctor might quietly say (for example) 'Your eyes began to water when you spoke about that' or 'You appeared a bit upset even mentioning your son.'

Confrontation

In some instances, the doctor can help the expression of feelings by confronting the patient directly, though quietly and sympathet-ically, with the emotions he is observing: 'You look very angry', 'You seem very upset just now', or 'You look as though you are going to cry.' Such remarks seek to identify the patient's feelings and give permission for their open acknowledgement, which is then likely to follow with therapeutic benefit. The essential first step in coming to terms with any distressing emotion, whether it be grief, anger, fear, or some other painful feeling, is to acknowledge it, rather than to deny or suppress it.

This confronting of the patient with the reality of his feelings should be based on what the doctor actually observes, and not upon inferences or interpretations, on whys or wherefores, which may be ambiguous and debatable, and therefore resisted by the patient. The essence of successful confrontation is that, when it is appropriately timed, the patient's suppressed feelings cannot be denied expression.

INCONGRUOUS ELEMENTS WITHIN THE INTERVIEW

In drawing together some of what has been learnt about conducting an interview, it can be seen that there are incongruous activities and that skill is needed to maintain the most effective balance between them. Table 4.1 sets out these pairs of contrasting activities.

Table 4.1   Incongruous elements within the interview

Facilitating communication	Controlling the interview
Listening in an unhurried way	Covering all relevant enquiries adequately in the limited time available
Avoiding inhibiting the patient	Keeping the patient to the point
Seeking accurate information about illness	Tolerating vagueness, especially from the elderly and the anxious
Endeavouring to follow a diagnostic pathway of enquiries	Being ready to divert and respond to the patient's disclosures and cues
Keeping a full accurate record of the interview	Not allowing the pen and notes to inhibit free communication

5 Communication by and during touching

Discussion of inter-personal communication would not be complete without reference to communication by touching. In all cultures, touching is a basic form of both social and sexual communication. Lovers touch to convey affection, and so do all human beings when they wish to convey, without the use of words, affinity and warmth, sympathy, encouragement, or reassurance. When comforting a patient in pain, a hand instinctively reaches out to touch. In the labour room, for example, one may quietly stroke the patient's arm or her hair during painful contractions. I have sometimes noticed in dealing with demented old ladies, agitated almost beyond the reach of words, that gentle facial stroking can help to reassure and calm them, allowing some communication to be established.

Here, though, we are primarily considering touching as a professional skill, i.e. clinical palpation, by which a doctor explores the surfaces of patients' bodies and the intimacies of their various orifices, including the erogenous zones, as a regular element of everyday work. What part does this play in communication?

CLINICAL EXAMINATION WORLD-WIDE

The routine touching of clinical examination is not a universal of medicine world-wide, but is particularly a feature of allopathic medicine within (say) the last 400 years and particularly the last 200 years. After the Renaissance, the expanding study of anatomy, pathology, and physiology began to provide the evidence on which clinical examination could be based and interpreted.

In many of the systems of traditional medicine world-wide—Ayurvedic, Unani, African traditional, and so on—physical examination, apart perhaps from feeling the pulse or inspecting the urine, plays little or no part, and the pattern of communication between practitioner and patient reflects this absence of physical intimacy.

It is an interesting reflection that the increasing sophistication of the biochemical analysis of blood, urine, and other body fluids, together with the expansion of ultrasonic and isotope imaging, magnetic resonance imaging, and computer-assisted tomography, not to mention interventional and conventional radiology and a growing range of other investigative techniques, may well be leading to clinical practice in which conventional physical examination will be minimal, or may even become extinct!

THE NEED TO MAKE TOUCHING SAFE

It has already been pointed out that doctors require a protective mechanism to professionalize the intimacy that is inseparable from clinical examination, and that they may achieve this only by virtually excluding the patient's sexuality from thought or discussion and by eliminating warmth within the professional relationship. Psychiatrists, in contrast, who are accustomed to verbal exploration of the intimacies of patients' personal and sexual relationships, are usually reluctant to carry out personally a physical examination of the same individuals.

How, then, do the sexual connotations of touching influence the doctor's professional touching and the part this plays in communication? For example, there is an obvious contrast between doctors' style when examining a child compared with an adult. A paediatric textbook will describe clearly how to obtain the maximum information from abdominal palpation of children. The basics are to keep smiling in a friendly way, to engage in reassuring, distracting conversation, and to touch with great gentleness, keeping the hands in gliding contact with the skin. That sounds perfectly straightforward with a child, but with an adult of the opposite sex might it not have the overtones of a caress? (Fig. 5.1.)

Anyone who has taught abdominal palpation in pregnancy to medical students will know that they have considerable difficulty in maintaining visual contact with the patient's face, still less in smiling while palpation is in progress. The intimacy of palpation is enough to handle, without the further intimacy of eye-to-eye smiling contact. So the student tends to frown down at his own

Fig. 5.1 Intimacy in the clinical setting needs to be 'professionalized'

fingertips (Fig. 5.2) or to gaze with a remote look of intense concentration towards a corner of the ceiling! Meanwhile, the opportunity for the student to convey comfort and reassurance by touch is neglected.

In any case, few patients are likely to relax their abdominal or other musculature unless they can immediately convey discomfort to the doctor by a change of facial expression. It is not enough to instruct 'Tell me if this is sore' or 'Tell me if I am hurting you.' Most patients do not want to make a fuss or a noise during their examination, still less to deter the doctor from finding out what is wrong. So there is nothing for them to do but tense up their muscles protectively and try to be brave. In consequence, the clinical information that can be obtained through palpation is correspondingly reduced. A considerate and sensitive doctor should therefore avoid touching any part of the patient's body, and possibly eliciting tenderness or pain, unless he is closely observing the patient's facial expression all the time.

Fig 5.2 Abdominal palpation in pregnancy. The student, feeling awkward, avoids eye-to-eye contact

GENTLENESS

Information is always conveyed by the way the doctor touches the patient. Many patients are apprehensive at the prospect of discomfort during physical examination, at the thought that rectal or vaginal examinations may be required, and possibly venepuncture or other painful procedures, perhaps an operation. The doctor's touch, even during a simple initial procedure such as taking the blood pressure, begins to convey a message, which will be one of reassurance only if gentleness is the unvarying rule. Similarly, the considerate gentleness and 'comfort' of the doctor during abdominal examination will reassure a woman who requires vaginal examination that it should not be the ordeal she feared. She will therefore begin to relax, and more information can be obtained from the examination.

Furthermore, if, as examination proceeds, the doctor succeeds in completing the vaginal digital and speculum examination in a sensitive manner without causing any embarrassment or physical discomfort, the *educational* consequences may be far-reaching. For instance, the woman will then not hesitate to return for a regular cervical smear; she will be less likely to book late in pregnancy for fear of a booking vaginal examination; she may feel more confident about seeking contraceptive advice or being fitted with an IUCD; she will be less reluctant to return to the doctor if she subsequently develops gynaecological symptoms. But that may be only the beginning, for the woman may mention how easy the examination was to her female relatives, and perhaps her neighbours. They too can be similarly influenced by the echoes of the 'message' of the original examination.

It hardly needs to be added that an examination that conveys feelings of embarrassment or pain will disseminate the opposite sort of message with no less widespread an effect. I have used here the example of vaginal examination, with which I am particularly familiar, but other examples abound. A painful, botched venepuncture, inconsiderately handled in the out-patient clinic (for example), may deter a patient from accepting further treatment as an in-patient. All forms of examination-contact convey indirect educational messages, which can influence whether patients continue to seek help and advice with their health problems.

If gentleness has so much to commend it, facilitating examination and helping to secure the patient's confidence and co-operation, present and future, why should any doctor be heavy handed? In some instances, it may result from lack of physical skill, but in others it can be a manifestation of the doctor's limited comfort and professional assurance, a way of ridding the physical intimacy of touching of any sexual overtones by making it a little uncomfortable, to be on the safe side! The doctor's dis-ease is further expressed by his frown and his 'Tell me if this *hurts*.' One might say, then, that the patient's comfort in a physical sense grows on the doctor's 'comfort' in an affective sense.

If the doctor learns to be truly comfortable with the intimacy of touching in his professional work, then genital examination can be used both for physical assessment and to help give patients with sexual dysfunction a new comfort and self-confidence in their own bodies, which can be an important element in treatment.

6 Caring communication skills

The manner in which a doctor communicates with a patient is influenced considerably by the degree to which he feels the need to remain detached from, or is prepared to become involved with, patients' problems and concerns generally, and with their feelings in particular. The extent of the professional 'distance' thus established is readily recognized by the patient, and in turn determines his perception of the doctor's role—of how much involvement he can expect the doctor to show.

CURING AND CARING

Because of the contrast between detachment and involvement, it is easy to generate a misleading antithesis between curing and caring. Curing is portrayed in this stereotyped view as a detached activity on the doctor's part, in which the patient is essentially passive. Caring is taken to imply involvement, a holistic concern with all aspects of the patient's situation. And so a contrast may be drawn between the interventions and technologies of acute medicine associated with episodic illness, and the less dramatic but sustained efforts often required in longer-term care, rehabilitation, etc. The first symbolizes cure; the latter, care.

The idea that such a dichotomy is inherent in the actual practice of medicine has to be challenged. It is quite untrue of family medicine, and even in the subdivided world of hospital medicine a great deal of acute illness presents in the elderly, for instance, and cannot be dissociated from patients' longer-term health problems. It is certainly also a false assumption that the doctor who does relatively more curing (or likes to believe he does!) needs less to be caring, i.e. that quite different attitudes and affective skills are called for in the two situations. Affective aspects of illness are no less evident and important in (say) the intensive-care area than they are in the long-stay geriatric unit.

CARING SKILLS

Curing is fairly easy to define (even if sometimes difficult to achieve), but what does 'caring' mean? The word is used in different senses in different contexts, but I would put it thus: a doctor who cares is not some sort of 'do-gooder', technically rather inept, but always compulsively eager to immerse himself in his patient's emotional problems. He is someone who has trained himself to develop and utilize, in his relationships with patients, certain professional skills which enable him to handle affective reactions with no less professional competence than he brings to physical or technical problems. The word C-A-R-E provides a simple mnemonic to list the main skills that the student should strive to develop:

COMFORT

ACCEPTANCE

RESPONSIVENESS

EMPATHY

Each of these skills merits detailed description.

Comfort

Comfort is the ability to deal with emotive topics, matters that may be generally regarded as embarrassing or painful, of which death and sexuality are examples, without becoming uncomfortable. This skill quickly communicates comfort, once the patient has recognized that the doctor is not embarrassed by the topic or situation. Consequently, the patient is not inhibited from talking about what might otherwise have been a subject to avoid although one central to his problems.

Comfort can apply to situations and circumstances as well as to topics of discussion—to disfigurement, to nudity, to things from which otherwise we might wish to turn away. It is by no means an all-or-nothing skill. Many doctors are comfortable with one topic or situation, but not with another. As we shall see (p. 67), doctors may be particularly uncomfortable when dealing with a problem that mirrors an unresolved conflict or dilemma of their own.

The following examples illustrate absence of comfort with a range of topics that crop up in everyday practice.

EXAMPLE 1

Doctor	'This is the third time you have been for a cancer smear in two years, Mrs Anderson. Are you afraid that you have cancer?'
Patient	'Well, um, . . . , yes. I suppose it's the things people say.'
Doctor	'What do they say?'
Patient	'Well, my next door neighbour told me that having intercourse during your period causes cancer and we often do it. But that's quite normal, isn't it, doctor?'
Doctor	(Speaking rather slowly and pompously) 'Well, of course you mustn't listen to things people say. Your doctor is the best person to ask for advice.'
Patient	'Yes, but it is normal, isn't it? I sometimes feel a lot more like sex at my period times.'
Doctor	'Well . . . of course . . . not everybody feels the same about these things. Now I'm going to take a smear when nurse comes back and you won't need another one for four years. Just go behind the screen and get ready for me to examine you.'

EXAMPLE 2

Consultant	'Now, Mrs MacLeod, we have examined you from top to toe and I am pleased to be able to tell you that I can find no sign of any physical disease, and all the tests have come back negative. I think you need to start getting out and about more. You have a daughter, born . . . let's see . . . she must be 16 now. You and she could go out together for company.'
Patient	'Doctor . . . my daughter is dead! Elaine started sniffing glue when she was just 13 and last year it killed her.'
Consultant	'Oh! I am terribly sorry!' (Looks away) 'How

dreadful!' (Pauses and hesitates) 'Look, Mrs MacLeod I'm going to prescribe for you a new and very effective antidepressant drug. I'm sure this will help you get back to normal again.'

EXAMPLE 3

Consultant	(To a young soldier who is recovering from disfiguring burns of the face and hands) 'Now, Robert. I think we'll be able to get most of those bandages off tomorrow for good!'
Young Soldier	'I'm not sure I'd not be better off with them on. I've watched the nurses' eyes when they're doing my dressings! Doctor, do you think anyone will ever be able to bear the sight of me?'
Consultant	(Turning away and addressing his remarks to the group at the foot of the bed) 'Sister, it sounds as if Robert's morale is a bit low today. You'll have to get his visitors to cheer him up.'
Young Soldier	(To the now retreating figure of the consultant) 'The only visitor I want to see is Angela, but she's not been near the place for more than a fortnight!'

EXAMPLE 4

Doctor	'Now tell me about your family, Mrs Bishop. You have a family?'
Patient	'Yes, I have three sons. They are 24, 17, and 16 years old now.'
Doctor	'Are they all in good health?'
Patient	'Yes.'
Doctor	'You must be proud of them! Are you a granny yet?'
Patient	'No. My eldest son will never marry, I don't suppose. You see, doctor, he's . . . er . . . a homosexual.'
Doctor	'Oh! I am sorry! I'm sorry I asked! I didn't mean to embarrass you. The other two are normal, I suppose?'

EXAMPLE 5

Consultant	(On ward round) 'Good morning, Mr Grimes. And how are we today?' (Note the impersonal patronizing 'we'.)
Patient	(who looks very ill and has obviously lost a lot of weight) 'I'm not feeling so good today. I keep being sick. Doctor . . . can I have a word with you?'
Consultant	'Why, certainly! What can we do for you?' (Note the 'we' again)
Patient	'Doctor, tell me straight. Is it serious? I want to know. Have I got much of a chance?'
Consultant	'Well, . . . er . . . we're not . . . er . . . exactly sure just at the minute how . . . er . . . active this little growth in your stomach is. But we've got some more tests and ideas up our sleeves, you know. So keep your chin up, Mr Grimes.'

EXAMPLE 6

Patient	'Doctor, my nerves have just gone to pieces since I lost my husband last year. I'm so lonely. It was so sudden. I still can't accept it. He was only 38! Now I'm terribly worried about myself.'
Doctor	'What are you worrying about?'
Patient	'Oh, just my health and . . . well . . . doctor, I must tell you. Since I lost my husband I have started masturbating. Sometimes I feel very dirty, and sometimes it really helps. Do you think I'm dreadful?'
Doctor	'Oh, come on now, Mrs Black! You're letting your nerves get the better of you. (Pauses) You'll have to pull yourself together. I'm . . . er . . . I'm going to give you some tablets to help calm you down a bit. You must get them from the chemist right away and start taking them three times a day after meals. Have you got that clear now, three times a day after meals?'

In each of the above examples, the doctor has revealed his discomfort with a topic implicated in his patient's problem. In consequence, the patient is unlikely to be willing to mention that topic again, either with the same doctor, or possibly even with other doctors.

Absence of comfort can sometimes be revealed in a subtle way, just by the choice of words. The use of a stilted euphemism can immediately betray the doctor's dis-ease. For example, the doctor wishing to enquire about possible extramarital sexual contact might ask 'Have you ever been . . . er . . . tempted from the straight and narrow?', or seeking evidence of alcohol abuse could ask 'Do you . . . shall we say . . . overindulge?' Or suppose the doctor initiates enquiries about sexual function in a similarly hesitant and stilted way with phrases such as 'Now, Mrs Black, is everything all right at home? Is the . . . er . . . physical side of your . . . er . . . married life satisfactory?' The patient is bound to sense the doctor's awkwardness and feel inhibited in replying. Nor is the patient likely to be put at ease if the doctor in this situation resorts to the use of sexual slang or false jocularity. Even a phrase such as 'your sex-life' is usually best avoided. It is too familiar, and its use may weaken the sense of formal professional correctness. It is best to choose a simple but direct and explicit form of words: 'Do you and your wife have a good sexual relationship?' 'Are you able to enjoy sexual intercourse without discomfort?', or in the case of an older person 'Are you still able to have sexual intercourse satisfactorily?' These questions are clear and unambiguous. When the doctor maintains eye contact while asking the question, his comfort with, and willingness to talk about, the topic are conveyed.

Acceptance

Acceptance refers to the ability to accept the feelings and attitudes the patient brings to the interview, without allowing them to prevent good rapport and communication. Sometimes these are feelings associated with illness that are liable to irritate or anger the doctor, such as irrational fear or mistrust, anger or resentment, undue reticence, inadequacy, or apathy.

The patient may appear over-dependent and feckless, unwilling to assume any responsibility for his own health, but expecting the doctor to produce some instant 'cure' for his ills. At the other end of the spectrum, he may be a critical intellectual, untrusting and always ready to propose some alternative to the doctor's suggestions. These attitudes may irritate the doctor beyond endurance. Also, he may sometimes resent strongly the time spent on certain patients' problems, which appear largely self-imposed: the fruits of an unhealthy lifestyle which the patient is reluctant to change, such as obesity in the glutton, chronic dyspepsia due to alcohol abuse, repeated pelvic infection associated with promiscuity, or bronchitis in a heavy smoker. In other instances the doctor may feel alienated before a word is spoken because of the patient's cultural trappings, whether it be the young 'punk' with shaved head and safety-pin ear-rings, the pretentious dame with lacquered blue rinse and podgy over-gemmed fingers, or the 'camp' style of some male homosexuals.

It is therefore important that the doctor should not be blind to his own cultural, social, and moral prejudices, so that these attitudes, which all of us possess in some degree, are not allowed to obstruct the development of rapport and trust. Prejudice apart, the more the doctor learns to recognize and understand his own attitudes and motives in his professional work, the more he will be able to understand and help his patients. Self-awareness is at the heart of professional competence.

Acceptance does not imply that the doctor should not seek in the course of time to change the patient's attitudes, if that seems a necessary part of treatment. It means that the doctor endeavours to identify *why* the patient feels or behaves as he does, and equally why he himself may be antagonized by the patient's behaviour. This insight helps to prevent the doctor from reacting in a way that hinders understanding and blocks communication between the patient and himself.

The patient's personal and family history often sheds light on his attitudes to the present illness. For example, a period spent in hospital as a small child, for (say) tonsillectomy, may leave behind a lifelong fear of hospitals, sometimes deserving the term 'hospital phobia'. Even visits during childhood to a dying close relative in hospital may have a similar effect. A relative's or friend's death from cancer can leave a legacy of obsessive fear. Sometimes the patient gains insight and reassurance when the significance of past experiences are explained to him. The patient may be aware of the irrational or unacceptable nature of his feelings, but unable to control them. The fact that he senses the doctor is accepting him as he is can greatly facilitate their relationship.

Again, it is common for the mother of young children who is unsupported through single-parenthood, divorce, separation, or widowhood to be beset by anxiety about her own health, especially when she is the family's sole breadwinner. Her awareness of the children's dependence on her well-being may constantly cloud her thoughts with irrational fear, and she may appear indifferent to reassurance.

The patient's previous experience with doctors may have generated deep distrust. If a doctor senses such suspicion or hostility early in the interview—if the patient shows a questioning, critical, or resentful attitude from the outset—it is wise to go over the management of previous illnesses at the earliest opportunity in an open way, to see if the origin of the patient's mistrust can be identified, and perhaps 'defused'.

As doctors become aware of the importance of acceptance, they learn not to use such trite and uncomprehending remarks as 'You are going to be fine, cheer up!', 'Don't look so worried, there is *nothing* to worry about!', 'This examination will not bother you *at all*', or 'Now, you'll just have to pull yourself together!'

Responsiveness

This is the skill of reacting to indirect or incomplete 'messages' that are put out by the patient during an interview. The essential element of the skill is not just in making the responses, but in the sensitive alertness that first recognizes the clue or cue, an indication that here is something about which more needs to be said, some affective topic that the patient might be reluctant to bring into the open without prompting or feels unsure whether it is appropriate to discuss. The clue might be an inflection of the voice, a hesitation, a gesture or some other signal in body language, or a more overt but oblique reference to a problem.

As was described in Chapter 3, it is often best to respond to such clues *at the time*, and therefore to diverge from the previous line of enquiry. Sometimes, however, it is wiser not to divert from what the patient is in the middle of saying, but to come back later to the matter that has only barely been hinted at.

Consider, as simple examples, the possible variety of replies to a common question such as 'And is your husband in good health?':

(i) *Patient*   'Oh! you will have to ask *him* about that!', hinting that 'He and I don't share much communication about personal things', or even meaning 'He is the sort of man who would be very angry if he thought I was talking to you about his health behind his back.'

The doctor might respond 'Why? Does he not talk much about himself?'

(ii) *Patient*   'Oh, there is never anything wrong with *him*', hinting 'And that's why *I* get very little sympathy!'

The doctor might respond 'Do you think he understands how *you* feel then?'

(iii) *Patient*   (Warmly) 'He has never had a day's illness in his life, I look after him so well!', indicating that 'We have a close and secure relationship.'

(iv) *Patient*   'Well' (patient pauses and speaks very quietly) 'actually . . .' (patient suddenly appears about to be overcome by feeling) 'I would rather not talk about that now.'

The doctor, responding immediately, might remain silent for a few moments, then leaning forward ask quietly 'Why, is it a big worry for you?'

Similarly, consider the varied replies one might hear to the question 'And have you always up to now enjoyed good health?':

(i) *Patient*   'Well . . . (long pause) . . . generally, I suppose . . . not too bad. I've never had anything serious *before*.'

The doctor might respond 'And are you thinking it might be serious *now*?'

(ii) *Patient*   'Oh, I couldn't say that! People at work are *always* telling me I don't look well.'

The doctor might respond 'And does that upset you? Does it get you down?'

(iii) *Patient*   'Yes. I've always been fit as a flea. Never had a day's illness in my life . . . up till *now*.'

The doctor might respond 'So what are you thinking about having to go into hospital now?'

(iv) *Patient*   'Well. I don't suppose I've ever had what *you* would
                  call an illness. But I don't ever feel well. I think I've
                  been suffering from "nerves" for years . . . ever
                  since I was a girl at school.'

The doctor might respond 'And what do you think happened then
to start it off?' or 'Do you feel other people don't understand how
unwell you feel?'

Here is another example, illustrating how the doctor's responsiveness can influence the direction of the interview.

Doctor   'You have had this discharge for some time?'
Patient   'Two years now, ever since the baby came.'
Doctor   'Does it make you feel itchy?'
Patient   'Sometimes.'
Doctor   'Does it have an unpleasant odour?'
Patient   'Yes, it does.' (Looks away, dropping her voice)
Doctor   (Quickly) 'What colour is it?'
Patient   'Well, it's difficult to describe, darkish I suppose.'
Doctor   'But is it white or yellow or green or brown?'
Patient   'It could be any of those colours at different times.'
Doctor   (Impatiently) 'You can't tell me what colour it is, then?'

Let us see how this interview might have gone with an appropriate
response from the doctor.

Doctor   'Does it have an unpleasant odour?'
Patient   'Yes, it does.' (Looks away, dropping her voice)
Doctor   (Responding to the patient's subdued reply) 'You feel
            self-conscious about it? Do you think other people would
            be aware of it?'
Patient   'Well . . . Yes . . . my husband certainly. When it was
            bad last year, he made remarks about it. I just avoid
            letting him come near me now.'
Doctor   'And has anyone, apart from your husband, said any-
            thing?'
Patient   'Well, not actually. But I'm always afraid that other
            people notice. I don't go out much socially nowadays. I
            never feel comfortable in company.'

Empathy

This is a commonplace of everyday friendly conversation. Empathic responses can be heard on every side, wherever people are communicating in a warm cordial way: 'You must have felt on top of the world!' 'How awful!' 'I bet you were mad with him!' 'Didn't you want to scream?' 'What a shame' 'Great!' 'Marvellous!'

These varied responses all convey a similar message: 'I know how you feel or felt. I could feel much the same in the same situation, and so I view your feelings, happy, sad, angry, confused or whatever, as appropriate. I endorse them.' Empathic responses do *not* signify that the speaker is experiencing the same feelings. But he is indicating that he shares them to the extent that he understands and recognizes them, and hinting that he could or might, if placed in similar circumstances, have similar feelings.

However, the doctor must keep in mind that each patient's feelings are experienced as something very personal to that individual. It is quite unhelpful, therefore, to declare directly 'I know just how you feel!' The personal quality of someone else's distress (or elation) has to be 'shared' in a more oblique and less presumptuous way. In the occasional instance when a doctor has indeed personally been through a similar experience to the patient he may, by revealing this, be able to create a basis for special mutual understanding.

Empathy, then, is a limited but positive response to the feelings experienced by another person, whether these feelings are expressed openly or not. It is not an indifferent aloofness or an open rejection of the other person's feelings, nor is it a sympathetic joining in the feelings. It signifies a middle way which nevertheless expresses understanding and promotes warmth between the speakers.

The use of empathy does not necessarily depend upon the patient openly expressing his feelings. The most empathic remarks can be made when a doctor is able, from experience or intuition, to sense the patient's feelings correctly even before he mentions them, and so demonstrate his own understanding of the situation. Such a spontaneous expression of empathy is even more likely to generate rapport and confidence.

Here are one or two examples of the way in which an empathic remark can influence the character of an interview.

Doctor 'How long have you been married?'
Patient 'Six years, doctor.'

Doctor   'And is this your first pregnancy?'
Patient 'Oh no, doctor! I have had a miscarriage.'
Doctor   'When was that?'
Patient 'In April 1976.'
Doctor   'How far on were you?'
Patient 'Oh, only 10 weeks.'
Doctor   'Did you have the womb scraped out afterwards?'
Patient 'Yes, I had to have a D&C.'
Doctor   'Which hospital was that?'
Patient 'I was staying in Birmingham at the time. I can't remember the name of the hospital.'
Doctor   'Try to remember it. You see, it's quite important that I write to get all the particulars. Can you give me *any* lead where it was? What was the doctor's name?'

The patient now feels inadequate, unable to help the doctor in what he obviously feels are important enquiries. But beyond that, the patient has had no opportunity to convey to the doctor how she feels about her first pregnancy. He has appeared to be concerned only with the physical events of the miscarriage, and oblivious to her reactions to those events.

Now let us pick up that interview again part way through, and see the difference when an empathic response is made by the doctor.

Doctor   'How far on were you?'
Patient 'Oh, only 10 weeks.'
Doctor   'Had you been trying for a pregnancy for long?'
Patient 'Yes, for about three years.'
Doctor   '*That must have been a terrible disappointment for you*!'
Patient 'Yes, it was like the end of the world! My husband was so disappointed too. I felt miserable for months afterwards. I suppose that's why I'm so worried this time. I daren't let myself believe that I'm going to have a baby.'

Here is another example of how the introduction of an empathic remark can open up the conversation.

Doctor   'Are your parents both alive?'
Patient 'No, my mother died in 1968.'
Doctor   'What was the matter with her?'
Patient 'I think it was cancer, doctor.'

Doctor 'In what part of the body?'
Patient 'I am not sure.'
Doctor 'Did she have an operation? Was it in this hospital? Can you tell me anything about it?'

Now see the difference an empathic response brings.

Doctor 'Are your parents both alive?'
Patient 'No, my mother died in 1968.'
Doctor (Pausing) *'You were only 12 then!'*
Patient 'Yes, it really was the last of my childhood. I had to help my father look after her when she came home from hospital. She had cancer, you know. Actually, I often think about her. I keep hoping the same never happens to me.'

Empathy, we see, provides an appropriate controlled, professional reaction to the patient's affective responses to illness. It not only assures the patient that his doctor understands how he feels but it *protects* the doctor, delimiting the extent of his affective involvement with the patient's problem.

The student needs to appreciate clearly the limits implied in responding with empathy. Those involved in the task of caring, *have* to maintain an appropriate professional distance. When doctors are criticized for their professional aloofness, it is often asserted that they ought to display more humanity. Indeed, humanity in dealing with patients is a declared learning goal of the curriculum in some medical schools. But the natural spontaneous human reaction to the distress of another person is sympathy—a true sharing of painful emotion (literally, 'suffering together'). This is a burden that becomes unsupportable when it is constantly borne. It is not surprising, therefore, that the phenomenon of 'burn out' [32] is liable gradually to overwhelm those whose commitment to the business of caring is too long and too deeply sustained, and who have not recognized the wise limits that need to be set to their emotional involvement.

The ability to use empathy effectively as a professional skill to facilitate communication depends on acquiring, through reading and listening, and sometimes through personal experience of illness, a more complete understanding of how patients are likely to feel in particular situations. Young doctors have not all faced an operation for the removal of a leg or a breast or a uterus; had a stroke; experienced an unexpected bereavement or a miscarriage; had a doubtful cervical smear; become diabetic; discovered they carry a familial risk of genetic disease; been told that they have high blood pressure, rheumatoid arthritis, Parkinson's disease, or cancer. But though one may know almost all there is to know about a disease, one can still learn more about how it feels to experience it. In this regard, various leaflets and booklets produced by patients associations and similar helping groups provide a great deal of first-hand information [33,34].

A series of Personal Papers published in the *Lancet* (1967–75), describing doctors' personal experiences of serious illness, provide another invaluable source of insight. Many of these doctor-patients recalled with feeling the distress they had experienced because of inadequate communication, especially of an affective kind, between their attendants and themselves. Their concerns as patients were often not recognized or were ignored, their anxieties went unrelieved, and they commonly felt in the dark, despite their medical knowledge. Although they might have had the privilege of carefully choosing their medical attendant, they often ended up thinking that the person they had chosen did not really understand how they felt.

These writings apart, each doctor's own clinical work should provide him with an ever-expanding fund of knowledge about how people feel when they experience ill health. So long as a doctor has an ear to listen, and so long as he promotes the expression of affect, he can continually add to his capacity for empathic responsiveness.

These four behavioural skills—comfort, acceptance, responsiveness, and empathy—help to equip the doctor to handle the affective dimensions of patients' problems with no less competence than those of a technical nature. The first two, comfort and acceptance, are concerned with the doctor's ability, when facing the patient and his problem, to *control* affective responses of his own that could be detrimental to communication between them, and hence to their relationship. They are skills that help the professional to control expression on his part of negative and often disruptive affective responses.

The latter two skills, responsiveness and empathy, are concerned with the doctor's positive professional responses to affect, by which he recognizes and elucidates feelings that the patient may have only hinted at. He learns to react not with indifference or aloofness, nor with effusive unproductive sympathy, but with a human response that is professionally caring and helpful to the patient but does not subject himself to an intolerable burden of emotional stress.

7 Obstacles to communication

THE PROBLEM OF TIME

The time available for an interview varies from doctor to doctor, and from day to day. The conduct of the interview is bound to be influenced by this constraint, but the doctor must not let the pressure of time affect his interviewing style in a way that inhibits open communication.

In general practice [35,36,37,38] and in some busy hospital clinics, the average time available per patient may be only 5–10 minutes, although a little more time is often allocated to 'new' patients. In a less pressured general medical clinic, 30 minutes or more might be available, and most psychiatrists prefer to spend a full hour with a new patient. In each of these settings, therefore, a different pace and style of interviewing has to be adopted.

I doubt whether it is necessary, or indeed helpful in a first interview, to declare at the beginning how much time is available. Such a statement might appear as an attempt to curtail communication, rather than to facilitate it. However, it may be a useful thing to do at a subsequent interview. Sometimes one has to decide whether to attempt to complete an interview there and then, or to agree and plan a second instalment with the patient, when more time may be available.

Obviously, the shape of an interview depends largely on whether it is a first consultation or a renewal of contact in the course of continuing care. For instance, in general practice consultations, the doctor already knows much that he has learnt about the patient in previous contacts. When a further interview is anticipated, the doctor has greater freedom to plan the stages of the consultation. He may decide, for example, not to conduct a full physical examination during the first visit; he may deliberately defer exploration of the patient's close personal relationships until a second or even a third interview; he may leave the exposition (p. 69) until a subsequent appointment. The patient should always be given an explanation of how and why the stages of the whole consultation are to proceed.

The doctor should try to appear unhurried and ready to listen, even when time is limited. Any evidence that he is short of time is likely to be spotted by the patient, who will then be less willing to open up. If the patient enters the room to find the doctor hurriedly completing case notes or pathology forms, or dashing through a phone call, or if the doctor hustles the nurse or, remaining standing, jumps straight to the presenting complaint, the interview will be constricted by a sense of haste. Richard Asher [18] put it well: 'To give a patient the impression you could spare him an hour, and yet make him satisfied within five minutes, is an invaluable gift, and of much more use than spending half an hour with him, during every minute of which he is made to feel he is encroaching on your time!'

But when time *is* at a premium, the consultation *has* to be streamlined to match the time available. In this situation, it is even more important that patients should feel they have enough time to describe their problems. The doctor's questioning therefore needs to be very selective. It is here particularly that the skill and experience of the practitioner will pay dividends, through his ability to formulate a diagnostic algorithm that leads via the least number of diagnostic steps towards a presumptive diagnosis. The learner needs to remind himself repeatedly that medical diagnosis is in very many instances a statement of probability, rather than the elucidation of an absolute truth. One could spend half a lifetime looking for certainty, but medical decisions are always constrained by time.

On occasion, an over-talkative patient will begin to take up an inordinate amount of time, embarking on a sequence of irrelevant items of gossip or introspective trivia. The patient may be a lonely character, for whom a visit to the doctor can provide a wonderful conversational outlet full of reminiscence, or he may be a born talker who turns every encounter into a self-centred monologue. The doctor, listening impatiently, may detect features of obsession or anxiety, manipulative fiction, or the stale smell of alcohol.

In each such encounter, the doctor has to draw his own lines, in a responsible way, between therapeutic listening and unproductive time-wasting. When he feels that the patient's rambling loquacity is seriously wasting his time, he should attempt to maintain control of

the dialogue without losing the patient's confidence. It may sometimes be appropriate to say directly something like 'Now, Mrs
Robertson, I'm very pressed for time today. Just try to answer my
questions, and leave it at that.' If the doctor feels he needs to be
more subtle, he can ask the patient to undress partially, which tends
to inhibit the patient. More simply, he can bring out his stethoscope
and make a show of auscultating the chest, or even put a thermo-
meter in the patient's mouth! Most patients are less inclined to
chatter if there is also a nurse present, so it may help to recall the
nurse if she has left the room.

THE PROBLEM OF PAIN, SUFFERING, AND DEATH

As already discussed, doctors need some protective insulation from
the emotional distress that can be generated by the pain, suffering,
death, and bereavement encountered in the course of clinical work.
They therefore need to develop an understanding of how these
influences, and that of death in particular, affect communication
between doctor and patient.

Although death is the one certainty in each of our futures, the
common lot of all humanity, it is something which people are
reluctant to contemplate or to discuss. Since, during the present
century, death in childhood or in youth has become a rarity and life
expectation has extended, people usually prefer to keep dying out
of mind.

To detach themselves from the painful feelings associated with
serious illness and death, doctors may elect, almost unconsciously,
to avoid uncovering what their patients' feelings are, and may be
inclined, therefore, to adopt a rather distant and impersonal attitude in clinical work generally. Specifically, they can often find the
utmost difficulty in speaking honestly with the patient whose illness
is likely to be mortal. In many instances they may have recourse to
evasion, silence, half-truths, or even deliberate deception. The
assumptions that underlie this behaviour run as follows. People do
not want to die, therefore they do not want to know that they are
dying. They could not tolerate being told that they are dying, nor
do they recognize that they are dying.

The consequence of this unwillingness to acknowledge the moment
of truth that mortal illness almost inevitably brings are usually

disastrous for the doctor–patient relationship. Confidence, trust, and rapport are likely to melt away, and cannot subsequently be restored. Often the patient's close relatives are taken aside and given a true account of the patient's condition, but made accomplices in the attempt to deceive. When they in turn later become patients, they already know how the pretence is staged. In this way a doctor can in large measure destroy his ability to reassure those patients whose illness is not in fact serious, for his word is no longer regarded as trustworthy.

If doctors are to counteract these tendencies and equip themselves to bring help and support to patients who face terminal illness, the first prerequisite is greater understanding of the emotions associated with the prospect of death. Much of this knowledge is recent, and derives from studies carried out in the hospice movement. Hinton [39] and Kubler-Ross [40] outlined five phases of emotional reaction that the patient who faces dying is likely to experience. Between the initial feelings of denial or disbelief and the eventual acceptance of what will be, the patient is liable to pass through phases of anger and resentment, bargaining, and depression. A clearer understanding of these feelings is the basis on which empathic support rests.

Those who are mortally ill may search within themselves for an answer to the question 'Why me?' In some instances, feelings of guilt or self-blame can arise. The illness may be seen as a form of punishment for past wrongdoing—the pay-off, the karma of oriental religion. These feelings can sometimes make acceptance of the situation easier for the patient.

In addition to a greater understanding of the emotions felt by patients who are dying, we now know much more about the need for the bereaved to acknowledge and express grief and mourning [41,42]. Too often the conspiracy of silence and aversion that surrounds death encompasses the bereaved family, denying them proper opportunities to express their grief. The reaction to bereavement and the pattern of mourning varies a great deal in different ethnic communities [43] (see Chapter 15).

In my own specialty, obstetrics, it seems particularly difficult to come to terms with death, grief, and mourning. Doctors and midwives alike are geared to expect a successful outcome from pregnancy and childbirth. Still birth is now such a rarity that we are ill prepared to cope with it. After a still birth, the grieving mother seems quite out of place in the happy atmosphere of a maternity unit. Her tears may be wrongly seen as an indication to administer a sedative drug. She is likely to be put into a single room, which staff may be reluctant to enter, not knowing what to say or how to comfort her. Opportunities to acknowledge and express her grief are thus denied her.

Gradually, the staff involved are learning to handle the situation with greater skill and understanding. A guideline from the Royal College of Obstetricians and Gynaecologists has set out the points of importance. Following still birth, it may greatly help the parents to come to terms with their loss if they are offered the opportunity to see and touch their infant, even in instances where there is some congenital abnormality. It can also be helpful if the stillborn infant is photographed, so that parents who subsequently wish for some record of their child can be given the print [44]. After miscarriage also, there is often a feeling of grief and loss that needs to be acknowledged [45].

These brief references to the distressing feelings aroused by death and bereavement provide a very incomplete account of this neglected topic, which is so important in its influence upon the practice of medicine. If the doctor is unable to contemplate death and dying with equanimity, he may erect for his own defence another emotional curtain that is likely to isolate him in a wider way from the affective aspects of illness. Death and suffering remain tragic enigmas of the human condition. But doctors have a special need to come to terms with these emotive experiences and not to allow their professional caring role to be diminished because they are uncomfortable when confronted with the prospect of death. Specifically, doctors in training for clinical practice should make it their business to acquire skill in the care of the dying and the bereaved. To achieve this they have to overcome resistances within themselves, while at the same time learning more about the physical needs of the dying: about the relief of intractable pain, vomiting, dyspnoea, or other physical distress; about the pattern of emotional reaction during terminal illness; about the most appropriate language to use when facing the insecurity of patients and the anxieties of relatives.

In Chapter 13 Dr Derek Doyle, from his wide experience at St Columba's Hospice, Edinburgh, discusses the special skills of talking with the dying. As skill is developed, it will come to be recognized increasingly that patients can indeed 'die well', and that doctors' and nurses' skills can be a crucial influence in such a situation.

THE PROBLEM OF SEXUALITY

We have seen earlier the basic requirement that the physical intimacy of clinical examination has to be professionalized, and so rendered safe for both patient and doctor. In effect, this means that clinical contacts have to be dissociated from sexual connotations or feelings which, in other settings, might be evoked by nakedness and intimate touching. In consequence, the patient can feel at ease and secure, and the doctor is not exposed to disturbing or intolerable feelings.

This neutralization of sexual feelings and reactions is not something affecting only the doctor. Equally important is the patient's perception of the correctness of the professional relationship, how secure he or she feels. This is influenced by the patient's cultural background. It will not be the same for (say) a former Pakistani villager woman as for a white city-born university graduate.

There is little explicit teaching in medical schools about how to desexualize the nudity and intimate touching encountered in clinical work, and the subject is rarely discussed. Perhaps the topic is thought too sensitive to be aired, and it is hoped that, by not giving the matter any consideration, it will assume less significance, so that clinical work will cease to have a sexual connotation.

Several features of the doctor's style and behaviour help to bring about this desexualization: formal clothing (in hospital, a white coat); a serious demeanour; formal correctness of address; a detached manner, giving no indication of any affective response to the intimacy of clinical contact. Conventionally, a chaperone is arranged if the doctor and the patient are adults of the opposite sex, and this tradition lives on, not so much because most patients in contemporary times expect it, or indeed feel more at ease when a chaperone is present, but probably because it provides the doctor with legal protection from any accusation of impropriety. However, a recent postal questionnaire among 171 male general practitioners showed that only 13 per cent always use a chaperone when examining female patients and 25 per cent never do so [46].

These trappings of professionally 'correct' behaviour may still not provide enough protection for some doctors, who might feel

over-conscious of their good name and of the need to avoid the
faintest imputation of familiarity; or who may find it genuinely
difficult to rid the clinical relationship of all sexual connotation.
Such individuals may, perhaps unconsciously, find it necessary to
exclude any thought or discussion of the patient's sexuality from
the clinical situation, and because of this wish not to be 'too
personal' the patient's close relationships and feelings cannot be
discussed *at all*. As a consequence, the patient may be seen in a
rather narrow, distorted perspective, which more or less ignores the
social context of his ill health. The doctor's lack of insight can, at
the worst, produce a situation in which his relationship with the
patient is not only desexualized, but virtually dehumanized. It has
become 'clinical' in the very *worst* sense of the word (page 7).

If the doctor does not understand the factors influencing his
professional behaviour, he may secure for himself a cloak of professional correctness, but only a very limited degree of inward
comfort. He may, for example, be at ease when examining certain
parts of the body that are within his clinical ambit, but not others
that are outside his everyday routines. A physician or surgeon
might be perfectly at ease performing a rectal examination, but
avoid carrying out a vaginal one. A male gynaecologist might feel
no qualms during pelvic examination, but could be less at ease if
the patient asked him to examine her breasts for a possible lump.
A doctor might feel comfortable so long as a female nurse is
present through whom a patient of the opposite sex can be asked to
undress 'Sister, I would like to examine this lady', but would be
rather less comfortable to have to say directly 'Please take off your
shoes, tights, and pants for me to examine you.' Again, a doctor
might feel reasonably comfortable carrying out physical examination on an ordinary patient, but be less at ease if the patient was
also a social acquaintance or a colleague, because then it is more
difficult to conduct the examination with an impersonal clinical
atmosphere.

If, in any of these circumstances, the doctor displays, either
verbally or non-verbally, evidence of being even temporarily
embarrassed, this feeling is likely to be conveyed to the patient and
communication between them will inevitably be disrupted.

In other instances the doctor's embarrassment may become
apparent when the patient voices a sexual problem directly. If the
doctor then attempts to evade the topic by responding negatively

with something like 'You'll just have to learn to live with it' or 'Sex is not the most important thing in the world, especially at your time of life', or even to dismiss the matter brusquely with 'Well, you know what your husband is likely to do if you keep on refusing him', the patient will feel even more uncomfortable and unhappy, and will know better than to refer to the topic again.

Patients may also be discomforted if the doctor, in a misguided attempt to put them at ease, adopts a jocular familiarity. Some patients find this threatening, and it can inhibit communication, particularly on affective topics. But if the doctor maintains an unhesitating comfort—not distant and aloof, not familiar and threatening—this is communicated to the patient, making it much easier for him to talk about affective topics generally and sexual problems in particular.

THE PROBLEM OF THE DOCTOR'S ANXIETIES

Another group of factors that can inhibit communication on affective topics between patient and doctor are doctors' personal anxieties, arising in the context of their professional work. It is not very difficult for a student to recognize and understand how a *patient's* anxieties may influence the way he behaves. A similar mechanism can also affect doctors. Van Beukesom gave an excellent description of the influence of anxiety on doctor–patient communication [47]. Following his account, a doctor's anxieties are liable to extend into the three main areas detailed below.

Anxiety about inadequacy or failure

When embarking on the practice of medicine, young doctors naturally feel rather insecure, if only because of their lack of experience. Confidence in one's own professional skill and judgement grows gradually and at varying rates in different individuals, but some people compensate for the uncertainties of self-doubt and bolster a shaky confidence by adopting a rather pompous distant professional style. An authoritative, brusque manner can help to ensure that the doctor dominates the consultation, and make it less likely that he is exposed to questioning that might reveal him not to be the clever, capable person he wishes to appear. As a consequence, he seems very unapproachable to the patient, and the aura of infallible competence that he carefully maintains makes it much more difficult for patients to expose their own emotional vulnerability to him.

It is easy for doctors to labour under the false belief that patients expect them always to have an answer to their problems and a cure for their ills. Of course, most doctors aspire to help their patients, and can therefore be reluctant to have to admit 'I don't know' or 'There is nothing more I can do.' As Van Beukesom put it, doctors who adopt an aura of infallibility readily rationalize their behaviour with assertions that 'The doctor must become the high-priest of modern times.' Doctors' professional wish not to fail their patients can unfortunately become a barrier to honesty, openness, and, eventually, trust.

The student is wise to recognize that he will not, as a doctor, really be expected to be omnipotent and infallible. All the evidence shows that it is not on their omniscience that doctors' good reputation rests, or their protection from litigation lies. It is usually enough that they are seen to do their best, conscientiously and honestly. If, at times, this means that they must frankly admit the limitations of their medical prowess, at least they can do so in the knowledge that their reputation for approachability will be increased—a more valuable asset in the long run.

Anxiety about patients' emotional reactions

Doctors can feel seriously inhibited from mentioning topics that patients might be 'touchy' about, including such varied subjects as taking more responsibility for an aging demented parent, previous termination of pregnancy, thoughts of suicide. Other questions that might need to be raised can be deeply resented and make the patient quite angry—matters such as infidelity, possible child abuse, homosexuality, the possibility that a skin rash might be factitious, to cite a few examples.

A student or less experienced doctor may not have learned the least upsetting ways of posing 'difficult' questions of this sort but, with or without this technical skill, may be desperately anxious not to evoke an angry scene. He may avoid this anxiety by never discussing 'personal' topics with patients.

Another emotional reaction from the patient that a doctor may fight shy of is the distress provoked by learning bad news. In an earlier section, we discussed how death and dying can be treated as topics too distressing to mention, though sometimes difficult to avoid. Doctors get considerable professional and personal satisfaction from being the bearers of good news (of cure, of recovery, of a problem resolved), but there are inevitably occasions when they must act as the bearers of bad news likely to cause emotional distress—tears, bewilderment, grief. They might have to tell someone that they are permanently and seriously disabled following injury; tell a couple that their infertility is absolute; tell a pregnant woman that her unborn infant has a major malformation. Because he is the bearer of the news, the doctor may, quite wrongly, feel blameworthy, and shrink from the task, or tackle it very awkwardly [48].

A further kind of emotional 'scene' that a doctor may seek to avoid is any display of strife or discord, either involving himself or occurring between other people in his presence. His aversion to conflict and aggression may mean that he is unwilling to see together, let alone try to counsel, two people who are at odds with each other, such as an adolescent and a parent, a young woman and her mother-in-law, or a married couple whose relationship is under strain.

Anxiety relating to unresolved personal problems

An area of inter-personal conflict can create even more intense anxiety for a doctor if the difficulty in his patient's life mirrors some unresolved problem within his own personal and family life, some painful, distressing circumstance that he is trying to forget or keep out of his mind, or even to deny. There might be disharmony in his marriage; anxiety or conflict resulting from his adolescent children's experiments with sex, alcohol, or other drugs; guilt about an extramarital affair, or an abortion.

Because of deep sensitivity about such a topic, a doctor may bluntly brush off any discussion of a similar problem affecting one of his patients, or attempt to dismiss the whole matter with a joke:

'Look! I'm not a social worker. I'm a busy doctor.'
'I don't think I have time to go into that today.'
'Well. You've made your bed, you'll have to lie on it!'

We can therefore contrast the different effects a doctor's own experiences in life may have on his professional effectiveness. Often the doctor's personal encounters with illness, disability, or emotional distress can provide him with great insight into patients' problems, and reinforce his ability to respond empathically to patients with similar misfortunes. If he gains the confidence to share his own experiences, this self-disclosure can promote strong mutual understanding (see p. 53). But if life has left him with tender emotional scars that have refused to heal, he may be professionally hamstrung when a patient presents with a comparable problem.

To summarize, the factors we have been discussing can and do have a big influence on doctors' professional manner. In different ways, they can and do inhibit many doctors from involvement with affective aspects of ill health. Unless these inhibitions are understood, and neutralized through insight and professional skill, the doctor is liable to maintain a distance and a lack of warmth in his clinical work that he may not truly intend, but that constitute a barrier between himself and his patients through which he has no keys to pass.

8 The exposition

Attention has so far been focused on the first part of the consultation—the interview—and relatively little has been said about the 'exposition'. This is the part of the consultation in which a doctor gives his opinions about the whole situation: the diagnosis and the prognosis; what needs to be done, or sometimes what little can be done; any medication to be prescribed, or any other specific treatment; and what action the patient should take [7].

The principles of affective communication are the same whatever the context, and the style and manner of the consultation are set initially during the interview. Because the details of the exposition in different areas of medical practice are so diverse, it is difficult to specify what is appropriate concisely.

Those who have learnt the art of interviewing will not forget their skills during the exposition! This is not meant to imply that the exposition can be taken for granted, but there is good evidence that, with better interviewing, patients hear and hearken to the doctor's advice better [49,50]. Besides promoting greater compliance, good communication is also likely to reduce the need to prescribe drugs at all.

If the exposition is to achieve its purpose, the doctor needs to be properly prepared. In the first place, he should have brought together the information on which the exposition will be based. This information is of two kinds. When the exposition follows various investigations and tests, the doctor must ensure that he has the laboratory, X-ray, and similar reports to hand. The efficiency of the filing and reception staff in the case of an out-patient, or of the house officer in the case of an in-patient, is vital in bringing together all the reports in good time for the interview with the patient. Sometimes a telephone call may be necessary to complete a missing item. It is most unsatisfactory if the doctor's conclusions and advice about the patient's problem are qualified with all sorts of ifs and buts because information that should have been available is not to hand. No amount of empathy can compensate for absence of facts!

The second kind of information required for the exposition is knowledge of what the patient has already been told. This is particularly important in hospital, where a variety of medical and nursing staff may have given the patient information, details of which should always be carefully documented in the case records (page 72). Without the continuity that this written information promotes, the patient is at risk of being given conflicting opinions and statements, so that at the end of the day he may have a rather confused picture of his illness and the plan of management.

In addition to availability of information, a further element contributes greatly to the success of the exposition. This is the doctor's skill in choosing vocabulary suitable to the patient. The form of words and choice of terms will differ from one patient to another; it will be influenced by their education, cultural and occupational background, and other factors. Terms the doctor may regard as 'innocent' and reassuring may readily create serious anxiety. For example, when a woman with a cervical erosion is told that she has 'just a small ulcer on the neck of the womb', she may infer the presence of serious disease, imminently or actually malignant, and be too alarmed to try to clarify what the doctor's words really mean. The middle-aged man with a sore back who is X-rayed and then reassured that it 'just shows some early arthritis in the spine', may associate the term arthritis with severe manifestations of advanced rheumatoid arthritis observed in a relative or acquaintance, and be convinced that he faces a future of crippling disability.

During the exposition, therefore, it is often helpful to ask 'Do you understand that?' and also to invite the patient to say what *he* understands a particular diagnostic term to mean. Only in this way can one be sure that the patient has a clear and correct idea of the nature of his illness.

WRITTEN HANDOUTS AND INFORMATION BOOKLETS

Even when, during the exposition, the utmost care is taken to explain matters clearly to the patient, subsequent enquiry often shows that the patient's recollection of what he has been told is incorrect or incomplete. This is not surprising when one considers how 'keyed up' the patient may have been at the time. Sometimes, the patient forgets to ask a question that has been pushed to the back of his mind by anxiety during the interview. On other occasions, he may have wanted to ask additional questions about matters of detail, but have felt he should not take up more of the doctor's time.

For all the above reasons, it can be helpful to make use of written leaflets to provide patients with supplementary information on a number of topics, particularly explanation and guidance regarding treatment. In my own clinical field, for example, such handouts have been a regular part of antenatal care and preparation for parenthood for many years, but they are of value in many other situations. At the time of routine surgery, patients can be given a leaflet briefly describing their operation, with an account of what the operation implies, the course of post-operative recovery, return to normal activity, and so on. Other varied examples of written material of this sort include dietary sheets, contraceptive advice, pamphlets about stoma care, information about male and female sterilization, recovery after a heart attack, and briefing notes for sex therapy. A helpful leaflet for parents who have just experienced a still birth has recently been prepared [44]. Patients who wish to know and understand more about their illness generally can be referred to books or booklets such as those published by the British Medical Association or by certain patient self-help associations [33,34].

9 Written communication

THE VALUE OF THE CASE RECORD

While this book is primarily concerned with direct person-to-person communication, particularly in its affective aspects, something needs to be said about the written material relating to patients—the case records, letters, and so on—and the way in which these ought to complement and promote good inter-personal communication. If talking with the patient is to include the patient's feelings and concerns, this needs to be reflected in the written observations relating to the patient's care.

Clinical case records, of course, serve many functions: recording the history, clinical findings and investigation results, the details of treatment and the progress notes, as well as bringing together the correspondence between doctors. It can be useful for a student to study a few old case records carefully, and to try to trace the course of events—what was actually happening to the patient day-by-day during the course of the illness. Quite apart from problems of legibility, confusing abbreviations, undated entries, and so forth, from difficulties in piecing together the results of investigations, and from tracing a coherent day-to-day account of the progress of the illness, the patient's feelings and concerns do not usually attain even a passing mention. Sometimes there may be a brief initial comment, such as 'a pleasant, helpful, well-groomed lady', or perhaps 'a thin, anxious woman, full of questions'. This may be all that is said in the whole record about the patient as a person, and such clichés reveal more about the doctor who wrote them than about the patient!

It has to be acknowledged that the nursing Kardex record frequently provides a more comprehensible narrative than medical case records, and, more importantly, it often takes greater account of the affective aspects of illness, of how the patient is feeling. The differences between nursing and medical records are no accident, nor are they a consequence of the superior literary skills of nurses! These routine written reports on the progress of each patient, drafted by the nurse in charge, are the formal medium for communication of information whenever a new shift of nursing staff comes on duty. They are a necessary consequence of the pattern of nurse staffing, with its regularly defined hours of duty.

In contrast, resident medical staff have, in past years, remained on duty or on call for long and often indefinite periods of time, with no regular formal handover to another person or team. Information about patients was then provided verbally through the almost continuous availability of the resident house officer in person, so that there was much less need for a comprehensive sequence of written observations in the case records.

Over the years, the pattern of medical junior hospital staffing has changed, and now regular rotas are worked in most instances, inevitably with a great deal of deputizing and transfer of clinical responsibility. Similarly, in general practice, doctors group together to share a duty roster during out-of-office hours, and the use of deputizing services is commonplace. But the pattern of medical record-keeping has not yet evolved in response to these changes, and the need to ensure more systematic, complete transfer of information when a different individual or medical team takes over duty has not yet been recognized.

Whatever system of recording is employed, it is important that the patient's affective concerns are identified, recorded, regularly updated, and kept under review. If this is done, any doctor who is on duty, and who may be dealing with the patient for the first time whether in hospital or in a group practice, is aware of what has been going on in the patient's mind and of his reactions to his illness. With this important background information, the doctor can 'tune in' to the patient much more effectively, and not feel a stranger. Similarly, a careful record needs to be made of what the patient is told, so that he does not receive dissonant or contradictory messages from different doctors. This information should also be included in the letters interchanged between family and hospital doctors.

10 Talking to children

A. L. SPEIRS

Many doctors other than paediatricians have to deal with sick children. General practitioners, orthopaedic and ENT surgeons, eye and skin specialists all find that children make up a significant proportion of their patients. Therefore, most clinicians need to learn how to conduct a consultation with parent and child with consideration, care, and understanding. This is an essential requirement if the consultation is to achieve its objectives. Some doctors are regarded as naturally good with children, but through training, experience, and patience these skills can be developed and improved.

Paediatric patients encompass a wide span from the new-born to the adolescent. Parents range widely in social class, intelligence, and cultural background. The doctor therefore varies his approach, his questioning and his explanation accordingly. Indeed, this is one of the challenges and pleasures of working with children of different ages and backgrounds.

FEATURES AFFECTING THE SUCCESS OF THE INTERVIEW

Ideally parents should be asked to prepare their child for a visit to a health centre or hospital, though probably few do so effectively. They should try to give a simple account of what is to happen: that the child is going to see a kind doctor who is going to try to help him. If possible, the child should be reassured that he is not going to be left behind in hospital, for though he may not show it, this notion can cause much anxiety. However, the vast majority of children are now treated as out-patients. It is very wrong at any time to reassure the child falsely simply to get him to come along.

On the child's arrival at the clinic, there should be a welcoming atmosphere and a cheerful receptionist; a waiting area used by children should provide facilities for play, and there should be an area for feeding and changing babies. In children's hospitals, the whole environment is geared for children, but general hospitals need to make more provision for the many children who attend them, and an effort should be made to separate children from adults not only in the wards but in out-patients and casualty. Long waiting times are to be avoided, as young mothers usually have many domestic commitments and the children can get very restless and impatient.

A consulting room regularly used for children should be bright, with warm colours and cheerful murals, without overdoing the latter. A small chair and table with toys appropriate to a range of ages and both sexes can be available. Sometimes a doll's house or some picture books keep small children so happy that they do not want to leave. Children aged six or seven years upwards prefer a more formal approach and are quite happy to sit with mother. There should be no unpleasant instruments around other than those used in routine examination, such as a stethoscope, torch, or auriscope. Doctors rarely wear white coats nowadays and so avoid a 'clinical' atmosphere that might intimidate a child.

When mother and child are invited into the consulting room, the doctor should smile and welcome them by name, offer them a seat and introduce any other staff present. Communication is best when mother and doctor sit near each other without a large desk intervening. The doctor should have his desk on his right-hand side thus giving him easy access to the child who will be facing him and close to mother on his left side.

PRESENCE OF OTHERS IN THE ROOM

Privacy is important in all consultations and there is no reason for omitting this in the case of children. Unfortunately, in hospital it is not always possible to ensure complete privacy because of the presence of nurses, students, or others, but mothers will accept these circumstances provided they feel their child is going to be helped. If, at any time, the doctor considers privacy is essential (or if the mother requests it), he can ask the attendants to leave. Greater privacy usually prevails in general practice.

It is very useful to have a health visitor in the room, as she can provide the doctor with background information from her colleagues in the community and can in turn feed back useful information to them. After the interview, the mother should be given an opportunity to have a further informal chat in an adjacent room with the nurse or health visitor, so that anything she has not understood can be explained in simple terms. The nurse can speak with authority if she has been in the room during the consultation, and this avoids giving answers at variance with what the doctor has said. The health visitor can later pay a visit to the home if this is thought advisable.

THE HISTORY

Information from the mother

Obtaining information from the parent is a vital part of the consultation. The doctor should proceed slowly, feeling his way and gradually building up a picture of the child, his illness, and the family background. The real problem may be revealed only when a closer relationship has been established. Prying at an early stage can destroy an attempt to achieve good communication. In paediatric consultations, communication takes a triangular form, involving the doctor, the child, and the parent, each giving and receiving information, each observing and being observed. As the interview proceeds it is hoped that the mother will gain confidence in the doctor and will confide more, especially if the doctor is interested and relaxed and seems to have time to spend. If the child senses that his mother is more at ease he will respond similarly.

Junior doctors are trained in the early stages of their career to work through the history following a set format, but with experience, they learn to modify their interviewing technique (see p. 18). An unstructured approach is more natural, and effective, leaving the mother free to talk in her own fashion with only an occasional prompting or lead question being necessary. New angles will emerge that may need following through, but still the doctor must remember to return to the mainstream of the interview and not forget vital questions, for example about the perinatal period and the socio-economic background. During periods that are intensely emotional, it is appropriate to set aside note-taking and devote all attention to what the mother is saying. The notes can be completed after the mother has gone.

Although the *child* is the patient, the mother is a key person. Indeed, in infancy particularly, mother and baby are really a biological unit. It is therefore essential to assess the mother also, and ask about her background, upbringing, and marriage. It can sometimes be useful to see the father as well.

Sir Robert Hutchinson once divided doctors into the 'wind-uppers' and the 'pooh-poohers', and some mothers too are like this, either exaggerating the symptoms or making light of them. This is particularly noticeable in the mothers of children with asthma. Here the doctor should be careful not to be misled but to turn for objective assessment to a peak-flow meter.

Perhaps the last question should be 'Have you any other anxieties you wish to discuss?', as there are often other unrelated problems about which the mother would welcome reassurance. These may be about something she does not wish the child to hear; if so, he can easily be sent out with the nurse for a short time.

Information from the child

Interviews proceed better if the child's eye level is at or even above the doctor's! (Only headteachers look down from behind a desk.) The child should be addressed using his own name and with a friendly smile and a soft confidential voice. Address him as an equal and in a manner appropriate to his age. A consultation is usually fairly serious, so avoid trying to be facetious.

A period of privacy with a child can be very revealing, especially if there is any question of psychosomatic or emotional disorder. A child will never tell you about non-accidental injury or incest in the presence of the parents. It is well worth while, therefore, to ask the child what *he or she* is worried about, as the child might have completely different worries from the mother. Histories taken from five-year-olds and those older can be better than the mother's! Give them a drawing book and a felt-tip pen and ask them to draw a dog or a house for this can tell you a lot about the child, and also often starts a conversation.

Consultation with older children

In recent years, there have been legal problems over doctors being consulted by older children without the knowledge of their parents, or by those at variance with their parents over correct management. The Law Lords have now declared that doctors can institute treatment for children under the age of sixteen years provided that the child has been properly informed and understands what is involved. Normally, parental approval should be sought, but there are occasional, unusual circumstances in which the doctor may be a better judge of what is best for the child's welfare than the parents. This increased recognition of the *child's* rights should be approved of.

THE EXAMINATION

The co-operation of the child can make a great difference, so care must be taken from the outset to avoid upset. By the time this stage is reached, it is to be hoped that the family has got to know the doctor and that apprehension and anxiety have lessened.

The child should be respected as an individual in his own right and not moved around as if he were a plastic doll to be physically manipulated irrespective of his feelings. If clothing has to be removed, this is best done by the mother or, in an older child, by himself with instructions as to how much to take off. No-one, not even a child, likes being undressed or being completely naked in front of a stranger. Underpants should be left on if possible. As soon as the examination is complete the child should be dressed again.

Any instruments to be used, such as a stethoscope or auriscope, should be demonstrated by using them on a teddy bear or by letting the child listen to his own heart sounds. It is useful to examine the heart, lungs, and abdomen first, as crying can seriously interfere with these examinations. Unpleasant procedures, such as ear and throat inspection, can be kept till last. Remember that tonsils can often be glimpsed without using a spatula.

A baby can best be examined on the mother's knee or on a couch, whereas toddlers are happier standing up beside their mother. There is no difficulty in feeling the abdomen in this way. Most children feel vulnerable and exposed when lying flat.

If any discomfort is likely, this should be explained first and assurance should be given that you will do your best not to hurt. Some children co-operate to a remarkable extent, but this depends on the child's nature and background. Even rectal examinations are usually well tolerated provided the finger is inserted very slowly to ease open the sphincter. The child should be told 'I'm just going to see what I can feel round here.'

Occasionally, however good the approach is, one meets with a child who totally resists physical examination and refuses to remove any article of clothing. The doctor should appreciate that this is not necessarily 'bloody mindedness', but that there are sometimes good reasons for this type of behaviour. Some such children may simply be fearful of what is to happen and one should respect this and try to allay their fears. Others may be manipulative or undisciplined, and here a firm no-nonsense approach may work. If unsuccessful, the doctor may have to decide whether any information that is likely to be gained justifies forcing the issue. This, in fact, is rarely necessary and to be considered only when there is a possibility of serious disease. In most cases, if the mother cannot persuade her child to co-operate, then it is best to leave matters and arrange a further visit. I remember a domiciliary visit when the child heard a doctor was coming and promptly locked himself into a garage at the bottom of the garden! I never saw him and the problem cleared up spontaneously after discussion with the parents.

REASSURANCE AND EXPLANATION

This is the most important part of the consultation: it is in fact what most mothers have come for. The doctor will have considered the *whole* child and the environment, not just the disease, and will have made at least a provisional diagnosis, not a collection of alternatives. If the doctor is himself unsure about the diagnosis, then he should be frank with the parents and explain the situation to them.

Parents want to know why their child is ill. There is a common attitude that when things go wrong it is somebody's fault, so parents often need reassurance that they are not to blame. They also want to know what is best for their child, so a plan of action has to be formulated. Good communication with the mother, in the type of language that she understands, is essential, although the doctor should maintain a professional approach and not descend to vulgarity or familiarity.

It is futile to attempt reassurance by saying 'There is really nothing wrong', for the mother would not be there with her child if there were not a problem she wanted to be resolved.

Many common diseases, Henoch–Schönlein purpura for example, have never been heard of by most mothers, so a simple explanation of what is wrong must be given. If the symptoms and signs suggest a psychosomatic disorder, as in a child with recurrent abdominal pains, then time has to be spent discovering the environmental stress responsible and what can be done to relieve it. Remember to give some explanation to the child, too, as he has a right to know what is going on 'inside his tummy'. The psychotherapeutic effect of these explanations can be impressive.

From time to time, it is the doctor's sad duty to have to inform parents that there is something seriously wrong with their child, such as mental handicap or a fatal disease. Although this is a particularly distressing experience for the parents, the truth must be told simply and clearly, so that they are not in any doubt as to the situation. The issue has to be faced. Accurate wording is essential, such as the use of 'mental retardation' rather than 'a little slow'. Being too gentle and kind will mislead, since there is often resistance to acknowledging and accepting the full extent of the tragedy. Therefore, as soon as the diagnosis is certain—as, for example, of Down's syndrome—the senior clinician should see both parents together in conditions of privacy, and explain in simple terms the diagnosis and its significance, avoiding extensive detail at this stage. He should quietly express his concern and sympathy. After answering immediate questions, he can conclude by letting the parents know there will be further meetings later. It is not necessary to go into a lot of medical detail (say, of the type of leukaemia), but it is wise to offer a gleam of hope where possible, since this can help the parents to come to terms with the situation.

There can be a great variation in response to news of tragedy, especially to mental handicap. One mother said 'Poor bairn, we'll just have to make the best of it'. This, however, is the exception, as the prospect of a seriously ill or disabled child is naturally a heartbreak to the parents.

ARRANGEMENTS AT THE END OF THE INTERVIEW

Before the mother and child depart, the need for another interview may arise. A visit to a hospital, perhaps some distance away, can be a wearisome business for a young mother with many family commitments. Further surveillance, if necessary, can often be carried out by the family doctor. Some mothers may express a desire for a return visit though the doctor may not feel it is necessary; if the mother feels the need for this, it should be arranged.

Occasionally, it is apparent at the return visit that the parents have not complied with the doctor's recommendations. He should not be upset or angry, but should find out why this has happened, as there may be a reasonable explanation. The home may be chaotic, the mother depressed, or the child quite undisciplined and uncooperative. Non-compliance is certainly not unusual and doctors should appreciate this.

Many popular books on child care have appeared in America and Britain in the past fifteen years, indicating that parents feel the need for guidance that is not being provided by the health professions. In addition, there is now a great number of voluntary societies dealing with specific handicaps, e.g. Down's syndrome, Turner's syndrome, cystic fibrosis, mental handicap, spasticity, muscular dystrophy, brittle bones, spina bifida, and so on. These societies all publish booklets and arrange meetings so that mothers can be better informed and supported in the heavy task of caring for their children. All this complements what the doctor has attempted to explain to them. Fully informed parents can help their children much more than those left in uncertainty or ignorance.

11 Talking to adolescents

R. M. WRATE

Adolescents, because of their particular developmental concerns and vulnerabilities, present doctors with special problems in communication. By and large, they are a healthy group; medical contact is more likely to arise as a result of psycho-social problems than from physical illness. Apart from the regular medical consultations associated with the treatment of chronic disorders such as juvenile diabetes, rheumatoid arthritis, sensory impairment, and so on, the physical conditions in adolescents for which medical advice is most frequently sought are glandular fever, traumatic injury, and pregnancy. However, the last two are often associated with psycho-social problems, and these also complicate, or contribute significantly to, the functional impairment of adolescents with chronic disability. For these reasons, it is important for all doctors to be aware of the common adverse psycho-social factors affecting adolescents, and also to have some understanding of adolescence as a developmental process.

THE ADOLESCENT PROCESS

Adolescence is sometimes seen as a particularly carefree time. For instance, Wordsworth wrote of the French Revolution, 'Bliss was it in that dawn to be alive, But to be young was very heaven!' For centuries, western European literature has provided rich illustrations of the memory or experience of adolescence, but also of the intense and ambivalent attitude towards it. For example: 'My thoughtless youth was winged with vain desires' (Dryden). Was Hamlet such an example? Caught between love and hate, between intense peer-group interest and the affections and rejections of his step-parent family, in some respects he struggled with adolescent problems more contemporary than those described in *Catcher in the Rye*. Many adolescents now grow up in single-parent or step-parent families, facing an uncertain future both in terms of family ties and prospective employment. Sometimes the 'Sweet wine of youth' (Rupert Brooke) is never so sweet as when it is mourned. But family malaise or repeated episodes of illness, perhaps associated with social dislocation or long-term unemployment, may be the dominant experience during adolescence; for some it may be the many years of selfless support they gave to a disabled parent or sibling.

So for many, adolescence may not be a romantic time, and the vicissitudes of life can obviously affect adolescents and their parents in equal measure. However, youth is envied for its assumption of immortality; in Hazlitt's words, 'No young man believes he shall ever die.' Such omnipotence contributes to the 'very heaven' of adolescence, and out of it springs the capacity for impetuous mistakes: 'Youth is a blunder; manhood is a struggle' (Disraeli); 'She bid me take love easy, as the leaves grow on the tree; but I, being young and foolish, with her would not agree' (Yeats); 'Youth's a stuff will not endure' (*Twelfth Night*). Adolescents are frequently impatient but in general they are also uncomplaining, and sociological studies show that few fundamentally challenge their family or adult values. Instead, the support some adolescent children provide for their demoralized mothers (e.g. with abusive or alcoholic husbands) sometimes seems unlimited, and is given at considerable personal cost. A disturbing feature of some care-giving by children or adolescents is that it is given without complaining. In general, adolescents do not seek out support for themselves except in acute crises—hence the under-reporting of deprivation, abuse, and sexual assault, and the development of 'hot-lines' and drop-in advisory centres. Arranging a medical consultation for oneself with a family general practitioner may be an important (and rather unusual) act of independence for an adolescent; it can also be a small sign of an adolescent in considerable difficulty.

Putting aside the external world of adolescents, psychoanalysts such as Anna Freud and Peter Blos argue that within adolescents' internal world there is emotional turmoil; even in the most normal families, adolescents are said to oscillate between emotional regression and emancipatory striving [51]. It is difficult to tell how far this applies to the majority. Although it certainly seems true of many disturbed adolescents [52], sociological studies of normal adolescents (in the UK by Coleman [53], in the USA by Offer and Offer [54]) suggest that for most their teenage years are relatively smooth and that maturation is accomplished with little difficulty or undue stress. Psychoanalysts and sociologists alike agree that during adolescence most vestiges of childhood are lost and an adult role-identity is gradually established.

Identity formation, once the *sine qua non* of adolescent theory, is now regarded as a complex phenomenon that evolves over many years. For example, gender identity is established in early childhood [55]; a youngster's sexual role-identity begins with hormonal puberty, and development continues over many years. Erikson [56], a prominent American psychoanalyst, argued that the roots of an adult work-role identity are laid down in early school life, depending upon whether a child's initiative and achievements were adequately supported. But later studies (e.g. Rutter *et al.* [57]) also emphasize the influence of secondary-school experience, the extent to which the family fosters an educational commitment, and the importance of the employment opportunities available locally.

Other aspects of emotional development are the growth of a capacity for intimacy and the ability to cope with being alone and acting independently. Without this, a person is neither able to trust others deeply, nor to relinquish their support. Although the foundations for both capacities are established in early childhood, the increased drives of adolescence (sexual, assertive, and emancipatory) and adolescents' wider social contacts offer renewed opportunities for the development of trust and emotional independence.

Adolescence, then, is not a single stage of development. For example, as all teachers and youth leaders recognize, 13-year-olds and 18-year-olds are at completely different psychological stages, though both are experiencing biological adolescence (i.e. from hormonal puberty to the full development of secondary sexual characteristics). Most children's relationships with their parents and other adults demonstrate an ambivalence that begins to emerge, sometimes quite suddenly, in early adolescence (about 13–15 years of age), evidenced by questioning, suspicion, rejection, or contempt of adult values and authority. However, by late adolescence (18 plus) much of the ambivalence has gone, and the pattern of values that will characterize their early adult lives is established. Early and mid-adolescent friendship patterns are often intense, replacing a youngster's close family attachments and providing companionship for exploring the world outside the family and school. With the greater emotional independence of late adolescence, less uncritical friendships based on a greater mutuality of interests are possible.

It is also important to remember that there is enormous individual variation in adolescent development. In part, this is attributable to the variable timing of hormonal puberty, and in part it is gender-determined (girls' biological and psycho-social development is about two years in advance of boys', and they are much more preoccupied than boys with emotional issues). Adolescents are extremely sensitive to this variation, and so early and late developers often describe quite different adolescent experience (e.g. Weatherley [58]).

Considerable variation also arises as a result of family and cultural factors. For example, neurotic family functioning, chronic disability, or economic dependence may all promote and prolong emotional dependence upon the family long after biological adolescence has passed. Adolescent questioning or rejection of adult values and authority is uncommon in Muslim communities, and in cultures where occupational and economic advancement is dependent upon family influence. For cultural reasons gender-role expectations in particular may vary and, to communicate effectively with adolescent patients and their families, doctors must respect and show sensitivity to these various cultural patterns. This is particularly difficult, but especially necessary, where an adolescent patient seems caught between two different identifications, that of their ethnic minority and that of the majority culture; taking sides may be difficult to resist, but is not often helpful.

Finally, to communicate effectively with adolescents and their families, it is useful to have some knowledge of the contemporary interests and concerns of adolescents, and the common expectations of them held by school, parents, further education colleges, youth training schemes, and so on. One is also at an unnecessary disadvantage if common assumptions about youth problems are accepted uncritically. For example, in mid-adolescence, sexually active youngsters are far outnumbered by those who are sexually uncertain, and habitual alcohol abuse is far more frequent than the non-prescription use of drugs. It is also important to have some awareness of contemporary trends as they affect adolescence, e.g.

adolescents' frequent involvement in part-time work in their last year or two at school, which increases their economic independence, widens their social world, and offers opportunities for the rehearsal of adult work-roles.

The first principle is always to recall that, despite their legendary existential dilemmas, adolescents are rarely solitary. Except for isolated and unemployed youngsters drifting through bed-and-breakfast or bed-sit accommodation, no adolescent lives alone in the full sense of the word. Those not living within a family may have long-standing involvement with a social work department or be supported by and well known to hostel staff. Schools, recreational interests, part-time jobs, or further education all offer opportunities to build up peer relationships in addition to those provided by friends and siblings. However, medical consultations are typically conducted on a one-to-one basis, taking adolescents out of their familiar group settings. Much of this chapter, therefore, deals with communicating with adolescents on an individual basis, but those who habitually work in this field are also aware of the advantages of talking to adolescents in a group setting.

Within social welfare provision, these group settings might be some form of residential living experience, or group meetings held in a local authority office or neighbourhood premises. Within adolescent psychiatric services, the most common setting is a family interview, which all those living at home, in addition to the patient, are invited to attend [52]. This permits an independent view of the adolescent's family, and allows family members to give their individual perspectives on the adolescent and on family relationships. For many adolescents, it is also less anxiety-provoking than being seen on their own. In an individual consultation, the adolescent or the doctor often feels stuck for words, but the presence of the adolescent's family offers frequent opportunities to re-direct questions to others, and to invite family views on the concern that the adolescent may have obvious difficulty in talking about [59]. This setting also permits brothers and sisters to volunteer often very useful information; sibling altruism rather than rivalry is the norm at most family interviews, however competitive or difficult sibling relationships were alleged to have been.

Adolescents often want to talk about their health concerns on their own, and may be reluctant to accept the presence of certain family members, even where behavioural or relationship difficulties are being discussed. However, there is little point in continuing with an individual consultation if it feels very awkward and seems to bear little fruit. In these circumstances, it is better to voice the need to talk to others or meet with them, and state it as a need rather than a request.

Some adolescents find it much easier to talk of their emotional problems in growing up or having to make the best of adverse upbringings by sharing these experiences with other adolescents in a group. A one-to-one consultation with a doctor can be quite intimidating, and it does not offer the opportunity for healthy adolescent identifications or so readily facilitate mutual problem-solving. Adolescents with chronic disabilities, e.g. juvenile diabetes, can benefit enormously from talking about their predicaments and adolescent experience in a group of similarly affected youngsters, where the doctor or other health professional acts as a group facilitator rather than as a problem-solver.

The second principle of successful communication with adolescents is that communication should take place within a relationship, rather than from a detached stance. Adolescents do not have the same experience of relating to strange adults as their parents do; nor are they accustomed to adopting the multiple social roles that adults have to take. In consequence, they may bring a freshness to their contact with a doctor, but are also likely to fall back on stereotyped perceptions and responses. They are likely to be particularly influenced by their previous contact with doctors and other authority figures, and by their experience of previous confiding relationships. For example, their perception of authority figures may be that they are assumed to act in arbitrary, unexplained, or insensitive ways. The success of previous confiding relationships (with parents, neighbouring adults or relatives, guidance teachers, and so on) will also affect adolescents' attitude towards a consultation. It is sometimes quite useful to ask about such experiences in the early part of an interview, as it will not only help the doctor become aware of these factors but will also convey to the adolescent patient the doctor's sensitivity to these experiences.

Some form of relationship-building at the beginning of the interview is consequently most important. Even a few questions about family, school, personal interests and career intentions, previous contact with hospitals and doctors, and so on, helps adolescents to feel they are being approached as a person. Adolescents are particularly sensitive to being patronized by adults, so this enquiry must be genuine rather than a ritual. Thus, the adolescent's perception of the doctor is an important aspect of the doctor–patient relationship; it is helpful if the doctor is felt to be a person too. An 'opaque' doctor (betraying little or nothing of himself as a person) will be perceived as insensitive and unlikely to listen, and may seem quite frightening. On the other hand, deliberate self-revelation is often seen by adolescents as patronizing or exhibitionistic. Thus, an attitude that conveys interest, concern, and egalitarianism without relinquishing personal authority is the important ingredient of relationship-building with adolescents, rather than any simple prescribed behaviour.

The third principle is that communication is more than simply talking. The talking should convey a sense of being related to as a person, and a sense of the adolescent's predicament being understood. This may be conveyed by the doctor taking some essential action as a consequence of what he has learnt, or by his helping the adolescent to make a difficult decision (e.g. about a pregnancy termination), or even by simply listening to the adolescent's predicament without being propelled into the sort of abrupt action or problem resolution that the adolescent's parents might feel driven to. Communication is thus about something being shared, about mutual involvement, and in the context of a medical consultation of something important being shared, whether it be a painful feeling, a frightening thought or health anxiety, or a difficult decision.

Communication is a multi-level information exchange; it is not simply confined to words. As Flaubert put it in *Madame Bovary*, 'Language is like a cracked kettle on which we beat out times for bears to dance to, while all the time we long to move the stars to pity.' Words are given added meaning by the grammatical syntax that governs their use, by the tone of voice in which they are spoken, and by non-verbal aspects of communication, e.g. facial expression, hand or body gesture, and eye-contact or its absence. Words may be used in response to some communication, or to block communication, e.g. by a torrent of words or by a direct avoidance or disqualification of what someone else had said. Communication may be largely non-verbal; for example, an adolescent may feel included in the communication between a doctor and his parents if intermittent eye-contact with the adolescent is preserved.

Adolescents and their families may find it difficult to put certain feelings into words; the doctor might convey understanding by an empathic silence rather than by words, although it is always helpful for patients when a doctor is able to put difficult feelings into words. This might be as tentative as 'I guess there is something very difficult/upsetting you're/everybody's feeling just now', or 'Would you like me to help you make a decision about this?' In each instance, the doctor is trying to put into words the unspoken concerns emerging from the interaction between himself and the adolescent patient and/or his family.

The fourth principle is that there usually is a symmetry to inter-personal communication. Direct observation of interviews (e.g. by videotape recording) reveals not only how people mirror each other's non-verbal behaviour during a conversation, but also how the form of speech or questions also shapes responses [60]. For example, information-seeking questions tend to elicit information rather than affect, whilst affective responses are most frequently elicited by questions framed specifically to evoke them, e.g. 'How do you feel about all these illnesses your family has had in the last year? And what was it like for you?' With unforthcoming adolescents, an interviewer is often tempted to adopt a multiple-choice type question approach. Although this can be quite successful in getting some communication going, the answers often mirror the questions in both form and content, and quite a lot of subsidiary questioning may be necessary to establish the validity of the adolescent's responses. Conversely, a doctor may discover at the end of an interview with a patient that they did not talk at all about an issue they had previously intended to cover. It quite often turns out that the doctor has unwittingly mirrored the patient's avoidance of the issue. Again, at a non-verbal level, it is more difficult to establish rapport and empathy with adolescents who themselves relate poorly; warm or engaging youngsters elicit warmth and interest in themselves from others, whilst a sullen or hostile adolescent characteristically evokes negative responses from adults, and it often takes quite an effort not to react in this way.

COMMON PROBLEMS IN COMMUNICATION
WITH ADOLESCENTS

First, from the adolescents' point of view, probably their most frequently voiced complaint is of not being listened to; adults may seem in a hurry or appear just to be looking for certain answers, or only listening for what they want to hear. The second most frequently voiced complaint probably is how often a conversation turns into unsolicited advice or a mini-lecture. Either of these situations would lead adolescents to feel they were not being taken seriously, and that the doctor was not interested in their individual viewpoints or any initiatives they may be contemplating (which may be true). There are five less common, though recurring, criticisms or complaints. The first is that of being patronized. Second, the doctor seems to side with the parents, either not taking the part of the adolescent, or colluding with the parents against him or her. Third, adults are 'nosey' (i.e. intrusive). Fourth, the adolescent does not understand the questions being asked: the words used are 'too big' or the sentences are too complex, or double negatives are used. Finally, the adults lack humour. This last point is important because humour is quite important to adolescents, allowing them to talk jokily between themselves about difficult subjects that otherwise would be too embarrassing, painful, or frightening to talk about in a more direct way.

It is to be hoped that, with experience, a sensitive adult would not keep repeating many of these mistakes. Even for a sensitive doctor, the criticism most difficult to avoid might be the complaint of intrusiveness, since a doctor's role requires an enquiring approach. This difficulty, and the complaint of pro-parental bias, can be minimized by making it clear at the outset of the consultation that the adolescent is being seen in his or her own right (rather than, for instance, as the troublesome offspring of their parents) and by emphasizing that the doctor is interested in hearing about things from his or her point of view. Adolescents' complaints about 'nosiness' usually reflect strivings for independence rather than paranoid sensitivity. They usually do want to put adults into the picture, but do not welcome the regression (that is, to say dependency) that they assume from their childhood experience has to go with it.

DOCTORS' PERCEPTIONS

The two most frequently voiced complaints by doctors about adolescent patients are that they are unforthcoming or that they are sullen and hostile. In either case they are considered difficult to relate to, so that little effective communication takes place. Even where the parents have predicted this sort of difficulty, it is wise for the doctor to check that his own attitude (in the terms of the preceding section) has not unwittingly contributed to the impasse. Where it has, it is useful to acknowledge the fact, for example by saying 'I'm sorry. I was in a bit of a rush at the beginning. Can you tell me a bit more about what is upsetting *you*?' When the doctor shows that an error can be recognized and admitted, the adolescent's stereotyped picture of doctors is countered, and this alone may free things up. Since most silence and most sullenness is defensive, the particular value of an apology is that it reveals the doctor's concern for the patient and his dilemmas, and for discovering the truth, rather than being interested in superiority or control. For the sullen or silent patient, it is especially important to build up a relationship before probing too much. If communication does get stuck, it is usually advisable to switch for a while to a more neutral line of enquiry, which can help to develop the relationship further.

When sullenness or hostility persists despite these efforts, it is usually safe to assume that it is a character trait rather than a specific response to the particular situation (e.g. because the patient has been forced to see the doctor against his wishes). Under these circumstances, the patient's manner should be alluded to during the questioning. The timing of this confrontation (see p. 36) and the degree of directness is important; for example, 'I can see you're quite angry. Does this sometimes get in the way of . . . remembering to take your tablets/test your urine/follow advice about diet', and so on. In each example, the anger is referred to as a possible problem *for the adolescent*, but this controlled approach can be difficult if the adolescent's negativism has got under the doctor's skin. Once again, it is best to acknowledge openly when this has occurred, especially if it has happened to such a degree that the doctor no longer feels he can evince much interest in the adolescent's views: for example, 'Look, I'm finding it very difficult to help you when I'm getting so mad at you—can you stop . . . drinking that Coke/kicking the table/talking to me like that?' This approach may be of equal value with a bullying or intimidating patient: 'I'm not going to be able to help you if you get me frightened of disagreeing with you' or 'I'll not be able to think straight, and that's no good to you. So can you cut out the threats?'

The persistently silent adolescent calls for a different approach. On the whole, such patients are much more difficult to deal with, because it is often difficult to tell what is causing the silence. It might be unhappiness, depression, demoralization, anxiety, or perhaps severe embarrassment. It might equally be distrustfulness or an unspoken hostility, and some adolescent patients give barely an indication as to which of these it might be. The best places to look for clues in deciphering the silence are in the history that is available, and in the doctor's own emotional responses. For example, social withdrawal and tearfulness in the presence of loss of appetite and weight suggest depression, but in their absence suggest some form of phobic anxiety state. Either condition calls for a lot of patience, which is usually not difficult to find, and the doctor can put into tentative words what he believes the patient might be feeling but finding difficult to express; for example, 'I guess you're feeling quite/rather unhappy/helpless/hopeless at the moment. Can you tell me a bit about that?' If from the history there are reasons to suppose the patient has difficulty (perhaps justifiably) in trusting others, this needs to be included in some way in what is said; for example, one might add to the comment above 'You may find I understand you a bit more than you would expect me to!'

If during the consultation with a silent, seemingly unhappy adolescent, the doctor finds himself becoming *unusually* irritated or angry, this can be important, if indirect, evidence of a strong unspoken negativism on the patient's part. Once the doctor has checked that his reaction is not some displaced anger of his own, e.g. with a colleague, another patient, or a relative, it is best to make reference to the anger as if it originated with the patient. For example, 'I wonder if it's hard to talk at the moment because of how angry you're feeling?' If the patient denies anger or asks why the question was asked one can reply 'I was just feeling that' or 'I just guessed.' The denial does not mean the doctor was wrong, and the patient may be relieved that the doctor asked the question, endorsing the disclosure of angry feelings. Further silences can be the truth. Quite often the adolescent faces being excluded from the family. Because of these problems, the veracity of the adolescent's account should not be doubted simply on the basis of some inconsistency or later retraction [63].

To help adolescents come to terms with their feelings of shame and guilt, it is essential to point out the universality of their emotional response, and to remind them emphatically that as child victims of adult misbehaviour they were not responsible for what took place. Guilt is to be expected, but it is inappropriate. Often it is also necessary to spend some time letting them express their anger with the perpetrator and their resentment that their mother or family had not discovered and put a stop to the abuse, particularly since, in most instances, the adolescent will have tried several times before to draw attention to the situation. The adolescent may also wish to talk in detail about what took place. It is often not easy to tolerate listening to these outpourings of feelings and memories, and the impulse to cut off the adolescent's account or reveal one's own feelings, or take some other precipitate action is often strong. In each case these impulses should be resisted and time given instead for reflection, which includes considering how the disclosure might affect the patient's future relationship with the doctor. For instance, the perpetrator may also be a patient of the same doctor. Perhaps of greater importance, it may be difficult for adolescents to return to the doctor after disclosing so much about themselves. If the doctor feels this could be the case, he can help matters by clearly indicating that this is something he would wish to avoid: for example, 'I know it wasn't easy telling me what happened, and I suppose you'll now have quite mixed feelings about having done so—I hope that doesn't make it hard for you to come back and see me next week.'

Anorexia Nervosa

Adolescents with anorexia nervosa call for a special approach, as it is easy to fall in with their massive, though denied, dependency needs. They resent it intensely if the doctor treats them as children by (for example) offering vague reassurance that cannot be backed up, or medication with no clear purpose, by by-passing the adolescent when talking with her invariably distraught parents, or by not giving her a chance to talk to the doctor on her own. Whatever the individual factors responsible for the condition, a striking feature is how often anorexia nervosa constitutes a developmental moratorium, or even a wholesale retreat from growing up. Emancipatory strivings for control then become increasingly channelled into anorexic preoccupations; underneath the anorexic adolescent's controlling behaviour, her self-esteem is usually very low and her identity fragile [64]. Emotional over-involvement and habitual conflict-avoidance are common features of the families of anorexic patients. In responding to the difficulties of the patient and her family, it is important for their doctor not simply to mirror, i.e. repeat, the patient's or the family's behaviour by reacting with similar anxiety-driven counter-control, which would readily stifle any quite appropriate but tentative bids for independence on the part of the patient.

Adolescents with chronic medical disorders

A major problem during the adolescence of many youngsters with chronic disorders is the struggle they have to establish a sense of self-reliant competence and emotional independence in the face of their ongoing physical limitations and their continued enforced dependence upon their parents and health-care professionals. The oscillating pattern of child-like regression and emancipatory striving referred to earlier is frequently seen in this patient group. Much emotional or behavioural disturbance in these youngsters centres around this single issue, even when adolescents are apparently well adjusted to their disability. During a consultation, the doctor's role may quite often be to reinterpret the patient's complaints in these terms, and to recognize opportunities to foster a true sense of competence in the patient. With these particular adolescents, the doctor's stance might be best described as a consultant to the Executive, enabling the adolescents to become as much in charge of themselves as possible.

The oppositional adolescent

Underlying, or indeed driving, the posture of rebellion and indifference to adult authority and values shown by these youngsters, there is often the opposite—they are struggling with very strong dependency needs. They become most oppositional with adults who matter to them, although sometimes they may treat all adults in the same way, as they attribute to symbols and figures of authority the characteristics of arbitrary inflexibility. Viewing adult power in this light, these adolescents feel that they can maintain their own identity only if they challenge that power. In general, therefore, these adolescents require a gentle approach. Where possible their outspokenness should be accepted without rebuke; their aggressive stance and comments should be ignored or turned by humour; and their concerns should be listened to with respect. Often this is the converse of what they have come to expect (particularly from their own families) and most of these adolescents respond favourably, their gratitude being unspoken but none the less evident. Any recrudescence of rudeness can then be much more easily dealt with; for example, by the doctor reminding them how much easier it is for him to help them when he is not being sworn at or shouted at.

Family disruption and estrangement

Although much has been written on this subject and how to deal with it by using family therapy techniques [59,65], comments here will be confined to what is particularly applicable to brief consultations, either with the adolescent alone or with the parent(s). In general, it takes two to have a quarrel, and parents often unwittingly contribute to the difficulties they complain of by being over-critical or restrictive, laissez-faire or disinterested, sulking, or in other ways undermining the adolescent's moves towards independence.

In order to understand what has been going wrong, it is therefore essential to get full and exact details of at least one of the crises being complained of, rather than allowing oneself to be flooded with complaints of a general kind. It is also important during the interview to convey to family members one's own impartiality and readiness to listen to the viewpoints of all concerned. Once the family members have been listened to, it is their turn to listen; if any advice given is then not followed through, they have less cause for complaint.

With some estranged adolescents and their families, the task is a different and often more difficult one: helping them gradually to accept one another's limitations. For a few, this may mean living independently, either as an immediate necessity or as a long-term requirement.

SUMMARY

Despite the many difficulties described in this chapter, talking with adolescents is usually rewarding, since most are lively, curious, and hopeful that their concerns will be taken seriously. Because they are in transition from childhood, their dependency needs are still great and their family identifications are strong. Thus, adults remain extremely important figures in the lives of most young people, even though at times they and their parents may doubt that this is so. There is, however, considerable variation in psychological development during adolescence, partly a result of biological factors and partly related to socio-cultural influences.

Previous experience of confiding relationships, both familial and extra-familial, are particularly important influences, and will certainly affect how adolescents respond to any medical consultation. Some may welcome the opportunity to speak alone, while others find this intimidating and feel at ease only if a relative or their family is present. In whichever way they are met, some initial relationship-building is an important step, and good continued communication is dependent upon a good relationship being preserved thereafter. This is especially true for those youngsters for whom it was the parents, or other adults, who were responsible for the consultation taking place.

A non-patronizing attitude and a preparedness to listen are vital. Attention should be paid to non-verbal aspects of communication, and to the manner of what is said as well as to the words. At times this may include relying on one's intuitive understanding of the adolescent, and scrutinizing one's own emotional reactions. Where possible, it is generally helpful to maintain an attitude of hopefulness and an expectation of finding positives in the adolescent. For example, just as most adolescents welcome sharing their predicaments with a doctor whom they would regard as a trusted adult, so do most adolescents respond well when of necessity the doctor in turn decides to share with them a predicament in which the youngster has placed the doctor; say, by wanting the doctor not to tell their parents that they are 18 weeks pregnant. Talking to the adolescent then becomes mutual problem-solving, rather than something that is 'done to' the adolescent.

12 Talking to the elderly

C. T. CURRIE

The past is another country, from which there are visitors among us. They are the elderly. For them, many things are different: money*, transport, communications, newspapers, public and private behaviour, even the landscape of the streets. Most older people have adapted quite well to the gradual transition from the familiarities of the period in which their attitudes were formed, but young people dealing with elderly patients should at least be aware of just how much change is involved.

People in their twenties today who are looking after people as old as the century should know that in their generation childhood death from infectious illness was commonplace, that the men could have been among the younger participants in the First World War, and that the women were among the first to have the vote. In their young adulthood, jazz was new, cars were rare, doctors were expensive and largely ineffective visitors to their homes, divorce was extremely unusual, employment was hard to come by, and housework was for most a gruelling and messy business. Whether as civilians or as servicemen and women, they have endured the rigours of two world wars. And to keep the generation gap in perspective, it is also worth remembering that the 80-year-olds of the 1920s were survivors from the early victorian era.

Generalizations about the elderly abound, but few of them withstand rigorous inspection. There is perhaps one exception, illustrated by the life of a distant relative of mine. Great-aunt Kate was born in the 1870s. A woman of some spirit, she was an active suffragette in the early part of this century. Later, when women drivers were still very unusual, she was a 'prominent lady motorist'. She raised a

* Two elderly women were overheard discussing the decimalization of British currency in 1972: 'They should have waited until all the old people died off before they changed the money.'

family and was widowed and re-entered local politics and caused consternation as one of a minority who welcomed a proposed Polaris base in the early 1960s. When she was 99 and still living alone in a bungalow she had occupied for 60 years, she became somewhat frail and accepted the services of a home help. When she was 101, she showed signs of senile dementia and became more dependent, eventually entering a nursing home. She died at the age of 102. If there is a generalization about old age, it might be that the second hundred years is tougher!

The diversity of the elderly is the principal attraction in being involved in their care. Any randomly selected group of old people will demonstrate a huge range of physical and mental preservation, of personality, and of life history. Most old people are easy to communicate with, a few less so. Barriers to communication are worth learning about, and the acquisition of a little understanding and a few basic skills is a simple and a rewarding exercise. Although most old people are well, the presence in the health-care system of a small percentage of a very large number—nine million UK citizens are of pensionable age—means that in most specialties many or even most clinical encounters are with the elderly.

ATTITUDES TO THE ELDERLY

Unfortunately, the education of health-care professionals does not reflect this demographic reality. In teaching hospitals, the older patient is often seen as some kind of marginally acceptable substitute for the real thing. Surgical wards and acute medical units somehow persist with an internalized model of a bygone age when patients had the courtesy to be young and the wisdom to present with only one diagnosis. The challenge of an inexorable shift towards the provision of acute services for an elderly out-patient and in-patient clientele has been met with puzzlement or denial of the reality of the problem.

For older health professionals, whose training took place and whose attitudes were formed before the rise of geriatric medicine and its incorporation into medical and other health professional training, all this can be particularly stressful. Uneducated in the nuances of presentation and challenges of the management of disease in the elderly, and bewildered by the complex interrelationships of the physical, psychological, and social difficulties of some elderly patients, they may patronizingly over-simplify matters by talking about 'social admissions' or succumb to the temptation of defending a specialty defined as narrowly as possible and speak and write indignantly of 'bed-blockers'.

Such habits of mind among seniors are easy for juniors to perceive and hard for them to resist. Interestingly, there is evidence that the most junior medical students have attitudes towards the elderly that are more favourable than those of their senior student and junior hospital doctor colleagues. It appears that teaching hospitals have at present a negative effect on students' attitudes to the elderly, although there is also evidence that formal teaching about the special needs and potential of the elderly patient can reverse this. In other words, if you know how to sort out the problems of your older patients, you will feel happier about dealing with them. This dissemination of a positive attitude towards the care of the elderly is probably the major achievement of the expansion of under-graduate teaching of geriatric medicine in the UK over the last 15 years. Unfortunately there is still a cadre of senior and dispropor-tionately influential doctors for whom there is no hope of educa-tion, only of retirement.

COMMON BARRIERS TO COMMUNICATION WITH THE ELDERLY

Dementia

Dementia, particularly in its lesser degrees, is common in elderly patients. Around 10 per cent of over-65s have irreversible mental impairment, around a half of them severely. About 25 per cent of over-85s are affected. Surveys of patients in the care of general practitioners and hospital doctors have shown that dementia is poorly recognized. Although the condition is untreatable, it is well worth recognizing and assessing, because some reversible confu-sional states masquerade as dementia, and because dementia, if present, affects the further management of the case in many ways. It is wise when dealing with an elderly patient to assume the presence of mental impairment until tactful but effective testing has confirmed or excluded it.

Because most doctors are in a hurry most of the time, and because patients respond badly to some of the more elaborate and less socially acceptable forms of mental testing (such as being asked to count backwards from 20 or to repeat gnomic sentences about a nation's supply of wood), the following test is recommended. Ask the patient her age, and then her year of birth, and then, perhaps with some gentle introduction such as 'And now, just to test your memory', what year it is now. This test is brief, non-disruptive, and has the great advantage of being independent of external verification and involving only a little arithmetic well within the capacity of most junior hospital doctors!

If a patient scores three out of three on this simple test, there is for all practical purposes no serious problem. One, two, or three mistakes, or straightforward incomprehension, have proportionate significance. There is no point in embarking on a detailed and complex clinical history from a demonstrably severely impaired patient. Other sources of information will have to be found. Dementia (or, less commonly, a reversible confusional state) has been demonstrated.

Undiagnosed mental impairment can cause great problems for the patient and all concerned with her. A vague but socially well-preserved old lady will react to close clinical questioning like a slippery witness, because she does not want to admit that she does not know. 'Which came first? The pain or the sickness?' 'What . . .?' 'But you said the sickness only a moment ago.' The truth is that she can remember neither the sequence of events nor what she has just said, and that time spent on further detailed questioning will be wasted. A few present-tense questions such as 'Are you in pain now?' and 'Does it hurt when I press you there?' will be useful in almost any circumstances, but time will be saved and frustration, embarrassment, and sometimes even risk, will be avoided by evaluating the mental state before almost any other enquiry.

The doctor assessing a mentally impaired elderly patient now has two additional tasks: to determine the nature and severity of the deficit, and to ascertain from other sources the information that would, in the absence of the deficit, have been obtainable. But to have recognized the problem of mental impairment and to have documented it will promote realism in further communication with and about the patient and in the subsequent handling of the case.

Deafness

Around 25 per cent of people over the age of 75 years have hearing difficulties, ranging from mild impairment, in which a loud conversational voice is helpful, to total isolation from intelligible sound. Many elderly people are embarrassed as well as isolated by the disability and may attempt to conceal it by a mixture of lip-reading and bluff. If a patient gives unexpectedly bizarre or even just excessively bland answers, it is worth thinking about whether they have actually heard the question.

Deafness slows up history-taking and can create or allow misunderstanding. It can also cause embarrassment, as when intimate details of a clinical enquiry have to be shouted aloud within the earshot of others. It is a simple and considerate matter to ask a patient if she can hear you easily. If not, there are several simple measures that may help.

The first is to speak in a clear and loud conversational voice with one's face in full view of the patient. If you shout, consonants tend to get lost and vowel sounds are distorted. In some forms of deafness, shouting can cause discomfort verging on pain. A loud conversational voice, with clear lip movements to assist lip-reading, will help most. If the patient has a hearing aid, it makes sense to find it and to check its setting or indeed its batteries, as necessary. Some wards and clinics have light and easily used amplifiers, with earphones or 'wand' earpieces, that greatly facilitate communication with the deaf. If all else fails and you have to talk very loud or shout, try to do so in a closed room, out of the main ward or clinic area, to minimize embarrassment to the patient and inconvenience to others. If deafness is absolute and the patient has satisfactory vision, writing short questions on a large notepad is time-consuming but worthwhile for essential information.

Dysarthria

Dysarthria is disordered articulation of speech. Language function is intact; that is, the patient can comprehend the spoken word and formulate speech and sound but has a difficulty, usually at the level of the pharynx, mouth, or lips, that makes speech slurred and indistinct. The commonest cause is stroke disease affecting lip and tongue movements. Missing dentures are a less common cause.

Various neurological disorders affecting the brainstem or cerebellum may also cause dysarthria.

A dysarthric interviewee is helped by patience, sympathy, and lack of embarrassment on the part of the interviewer. Persistence will be rewarded as the patient's particular problems with articulation become more familiar and speech becomes gradually more comprehensible. Where appropriate, finding the lost false teeth is an obvious and helpful thing to do, and will be much appreciated.

Dysphasia

Dysphasia is an abnormality of language function usually caused by stroke damage to the left hemisphere. Around two-thirds of patients with right-sided weakness due to stroke show some evidence of dysphasia. In most cases, both receptive and expressive language functions are affected to some degree, i.e. the patient has difficulty both with deciphering sound into meaning and with encoding meaning into words. Since major loss of language can occur with good cognitive preservation, dysphasia can be a very distressing experience for the patient, who is aware of his world yet out of communication with it. Perhaps most distressing is the plight of the patient with a predominantly expressive dysphasia who is assumed also to be incapable of understanding speech. To be talked about, perhaps unsympathetically, by medical and nursing staff unaware that everything they say is being fully understood, could be a hideous experience for an alert and cognitively intact patient, combining anguish, frustration, and resentment. It is kindest and safest to assume understanding until the facts have been determined.

The approach to the dysphasic patient is at first diagnostic: which language functions have been affected, and to what degree; and what, if any, cognitive impairment is also present? An alert-looking patient, behaving appropriately to his or her circumstances, is likely to be quite well preserved mentally even if he or she cannot utter a word. Many smile and nod as though to initiate a wordless encounter. Polite greetings—'Hello, good morning', etc., are visibly appreciated. Receptive function can be assessed quickly and reliably in the patient who cannot speak by asking him or her to perform a simple action such as putting out the tongue or raising the left hand. It is surprising how often that kind of request, intended to test purely language function, is spoiled for its true purpose by the inclusion of some non-verbal cue. A sympathetically phrased question about language function, such as 'Is it that you know what you want to say but can't put it into words?' may prompt an emphatic but wordless agreement, often also demonstrating relief that someone (at last?) knows how the patient feels.

The unlikeable elderly patient

Not all elderly patients are approachable, personable, and easy to get on with, and any realistic account of the problems of communicating with the elderly should recognize this. The rational handling of an encounter with an unlikeable patient begins with the recognition of one's own reactions. Only by being open to one's own less admissible feelings is it possible to handle them and remain both in control of oneself and helpful to the patient. The less attractive patient, the unpleasant patient, and the patient who is frankly not far short of ghastly are all still patients first and foremost, in need of care, assessment and management, and, whatever one's initial reaction, just as much part of one's job as their less repellent fellows!

There is no doubt that unattractive patients are at risk for certain misfortunes. When doctors are busy, they are more likely to be left to the last. If it is possible to delegate, they will end up as the immediate responsibility of the most junior member of the team. In the day-to-day life of the ward, they become isolated and perhaps the recipients of less preferential nursing care.

The first step, then, in dealing with the unlikeable patient is to be aware of one's own reaction. Thereafter, the trick is to detach oneself a little from one's reaction, to work out why it is the patient seems unpleasant, and to proceed on the basis that the resulting information is an integral part of the assessment and perhaps also of some clinical significance.

Health professionals are for the most part reared in the traditions of middle-class cleanliness. A dirty patient, visually unpleasant and perhaps also malodorous, is more difficult for us to deal with than a clean one. It is tempting to back off, or to adopt a more abrupt or even a judgemental attitude. (One of my contemporaries in a casualty job used to ask such patients when they last had a bath, and sometimes even enquire solemnly when they were last in jail!) To retreat is contrary to the conditioning and instinct to care, and sets up anxiety. To be harsh is to betray trust or, in some cases, simply to reinforce previous low expectations on the part of the patient. Negligence that occurs because the patient is dirty and therefore escapes thorough examination is, of course, unforgivable. We can do better.

The key to preserving calmness and efficiency in relation to the dirty patient is to develop an active and enquiring attitude towards the problem of dirt. Why is the patient dirty? Is the dirt acute or chronic? The significance of ingrained grime, black-bordered fingernails, and long curly toenails is very different from that of a single episode of faecal incontinence. In the former case, self-neglect is likely to be related to dementia. Because of mental impairment, the patient has lost the insight and self-care capacity that keeps most of us fairly clean. Brief mental testing is the next step. In the latter case, it may be that an old lady has taken her laxative, fallen, broken her hip, lain overnight in fear and pain, and in the morning endured the humiliation of the first episode of incontinence she has experienced for seven or eight decades. The clinical significance of her offensive state, the result of temporary helplessness, is very different.

The same approach can be applied equally usefully to other components of unlikeability. The first step is to recognize one's emotions; the next is to identify just what it is that is upsetting about the patient; the third is to understand that identified factor in terms of its clinical significance. Thus, irritants are neutralized by turning them into more information about the patient, for further assessment and action as necessary.

Other presentations of dementia can be equally irritating or repulsive. There are old people with severe mental impairment who are almost 'professionally old', coming across as vain and repetitious and saying things like 'I'm 93 and I'm wonderful for my age' several times over a few minutes. They may well be vain, with little to be vain about. They are a lot more repetitious than they think they are, because they cannot recall having made their main conversational contribution only a few minutes or seconds before. Again, simple mental testing will objectify the problem and a moment's reflection will greatly increase one's sympathy for the patient's regular carers.

Another frequently unlikeable patient is the undiagnosed depressive, particularly one who is hypochondriacal and polysymptomatic. Many of these patients have previous adverse experience of medicine, low expectations, and high anxiety, all of which further diminish the prospects of an easy encounter. The moaning old woman with a sore back may have been seen in orthopaedic outpatients, have been found to have arthritis to a degree unremarkable for her age, and been given a corset that did not help much. Other minor chronic symptoms may have taken her to other single-system clinics, and she may be on a great many medications. She pours out a litany of luridly described phenomena which bear little relation to what we read of in textbooks. She answers simple questions with psychotic intensity: 'Do you have a headache?' 'Yes! Like a giant banging nails into my head.' 'Do you get indigestion?' 'Yes . . . Like wee red-hot golf balls jooglin' aboot in my stomach.'

A good way of remaining calm through such an interview is to write down as much as possible verbatim. The cumulative miseries crowded on the page are virtually diagnostic. It is easy to see why such patients are unpopular and why they are passed from clinic to clinic, but a few of the key questions concerning a possible depressive illness will take the case a lot further. Yes, the patient sleeps badly and wakes early. Yes, her mood is low and sometimes she wishes she were dead. She has depression and needs a trial of medication rather than exhaustive investigation of each and every symptom. An unlikeable patient has been transformed to one with a single, highly treatable illness!

The patient has benefited and so has the doctor. Such an active and diagnostic approach to the unlikeable patient is in everyone's interest. The guilt of delay or delegation can be avoided. A potentially frustrating, muddled encounter, which could have left the doctor feeling angry and impotent, can be transformed into an intellectually and professionally satisfying part of his or her work. Most of us would rather help patients than feel angry with them or helpless about their problems. Broadening one's clinical assessment to include the unpalatable is not simply good practical medicine, it is enlightened self-interest.

13 Talking to the dying patient
D. DOYLE

Those who are dying, contrary to what one might expect, seldom want their diagnosis discussed or repeatedly explained. But they *do* ask, in one way or another, for confirmation that they are dying; they are then ready to tackle the business in hand, that of living out what is left of life with minimal suffering, with a dignity that is defined by them and respected by their attendants, and with an unclouded mind. As death approaches, whether they are young or old, they seem to invite the doctors and nurses caring for them to change their roles from 'professional advisers and attendants' to intimate companions on the loneliest journey a human being ever takes.

Some years ago, I and a nursing colleague visited a woman at her doctor's request. She had advanced oesophageal carcinoma with considerable pain and almost total dysphagia. As is my custom, I did not immediately take a history, but rather asked the patient in what way she felt I could help her: 'Ease my pain, show me what I can eat, and reassure me that you will always answer my questions honestly. I must be fit enough to finish some unfinished business.'

Some weeks later, so frail that she could no longer manage at home, she was admitted to the hospice where, again, she was asked the same question: 'In what way can I be of service to you?' Surprisingly, she replied with a question: 'Do you know what a platform ticket is?' She proceeded to explain that she expected to need a kindly companion in the near future. 'I feel as though I am on a railway platform, bags packed, a single ticket in my pocket and (just like British Rail!) my train is a trifle late. As if I had studied the travel brochures, I am excited about where I am going because it sounds so lovely but, of course, I haven't actually met anyone who has ever been there and I can't help feeling a bit apprehensive. As I wait here I would like someone to talk to, someone to advise me and possibly provide a bit of reassurance but, most of all, I just want a companion because I am finding it all a bit lonely. Will you get a platform ticket, doctor?'

It became a routine to stop at her bed and ask if it was time to buy the platform ticket, with always the same reply, 'No, so long as you know when to get it!' One day, scarcely looking any different, she called over and whispered that her train was coming in. I sat with her, holding her hand and marvelling that conversation seemed unnecessary, until she said 'Thank you for being with me—you can't come any further but I am no longer afraid or lonely', and shortly afterwards she died.

That vignette says much from which we can learn, though admittedly she was exceptional in being so articulate (and colourful) as well as so trusting.

'TELLING' OR CONFIRMING

Doctors involved in the care of the dying are often surprised at how much many patients know about their diagnosis. Many have already been given information skilfully by colleagues, particularly if they are younger patients who must be able to give informed consent and willing co-operation for what, in the case of cancer patients, may be protracted regimens of surgery, radiotherapy, and chemotherapy. An equal number, however, have no recollection of being informed but have deduced the sinister prognosis from the changed attitude of their medical attendants, the altered pace of treatment, the whispered conversations outside the bedroom, the painful embarrassment of loved ones, and their ever-worsening physical health in spite of so much care and attention.

Rarely does the doctor find himself formally spelling out the diagnosis, but rather *confirming* the patient's suspicions, which often were aroused even before help was first sought. But the doctor is often expected to explain the cause and the significance of the symptoms—not because they are seen as diagnostic pointers, but as indicators of possible new problems or the source of fresh fears. Dysphagia is feared, not because it reminds the patient of the carcinoma he has discovered he harbours, but as a cause of choking or slow starvation. It is not so much the patient's bronchogenic carcinoma that needs an explanation, but whether the dyspnoea will lead to suffocation, or whether the copious sweating means he also has an infectious condition. He wants to know whether his 'muddledness' is normal or the herald of insanity; whether his weakness is the onset of paralysis; or whether the fleck of blood in the sputum is a forerunner to catastrophic haemorrhage.

He welcomes an invitation to speak of anything that troubles him, however trivial it may sound. He does not expect a new prescription for each symptom, but only some evidence of the doctor's genuine interest in how he feels. While the greeting 'How is the pain today?' may elicit an answer gratifying for the doctor who has controlled the pain effectively, the patient would usually much prefer to be asked 'How are *you* today?', so that he can speak about *anything* that is troubling him, even if the doctor seems inept at dealing with his concerns.

ACTIVE LISTENING

The doctor, with his fund of knowledge and ready answers, may find it disconcerting when he is expected to listen rather than expound, to be inactive when he would be more comfortable writing out a prescription or ordering further (often unnecessary) investigations. At all stages of his professional life he will be surprised at how often he is remembered as being 'helpful' or 'reassuring' when he recollects only sitting, listening, and perhaps feeling utterly helpless.

Few people are so conscious of taking up the time of others as those who have less of it remaining for themselves. Whereas the doctor may fear that caring for the dying 'will demand so much time', he is likely to find that the dying are not demanding, and as death approaches ask less and less of their attendants and companions and are usually considerate to the point of embarrassment.

'HOW LONG, DOCTOR?'

Two aspects of this caring 'ministry' (for such it is) may frighten the most experienced doctor. The first is the way in which patients ask for a prognosis ('Though I know, of course, you can't give that, doctor') and then reinterpret whatever was said. 'Many weeks' is seen as less than eight because otherwise the doctor would surely have said 'two months'. 'Many, many months' may be interpreted as less than a year or even six months because it is thought that otherwise the doctor would have related it to Christmas or the summer, and so on. Nothing, however, is more damaging and upsetting than giving a ridiculously vague prognosis such as 'two months to two years'. Invariably the patient and family latch on to the more optimistic one and then wonder what has gone wrong and who is to blame when it turns out to be dramatically less favourable.

The other problem arises when questions of faith are raised, often thereby challenging the doctor to examine his own beliefs or philosophy, which, unlike the patient, he may not have even begun to formulate. His professional training may have taught him to regard this as such an intensely personal, private area of life as to be almost a taboo subject, and his relationship as one in which he must never be seen to proselytize or impose his views. On the other hand, since he is now regarded as a friend and companion, he should feel comfortable enough to let the patient express the whole range of emotions from anger to serenity, despair to hope. Sharing one's feelings about life, death, God, and love is right and proper within such a close and sensitive relationship.

So far, as will have become obvious, we have been describing somewhat unexpected reactions and questions that may surprise the doctor.

The terminally ill patient principally seeks confirmation of what is happening and seems more concerned about the manner of his 'dying' than 'death' itself. Although he dwells more on the quality of his present life than on thoughts of the life to come, he may, by alluding to matters of faith or philosophy, embarrass the doctor, whom he now treats, perhaps without realizing it, more as a trusted confidant than a respected professional adviser.

PROTECTING THE DOCTOR

The doctor is likely to be even more surprised when he realizes how much he is being protected by the patient. Not only is his busy professional and social life respected, but very often the patient engages in subtle deception as much for the sake of the doctor as for anyone else's. How often I have been called to see a patient by a colleague and asked the patient whether he knows and understands what is the matter with him, only to have the patient look around him to make sure no-one can overhear and then say 'I am being treated for bronchitis but actually I have cancer! Promise me you won't tell my doctor I have found out—he has been so kind and considerate I would hate him to be hurt, or upset that I found out what he was trying to shield me from!' On other occasions, when a slight change in medication is being considered, the patient will say 'I hope my doctor won't feel I am not pleased with all he has done—I would never want to disappoint him.'

This same unselfish consideration for others usually extends to loved ones also. The patient who finds it both easy and helpful to chat with his doctor about every detail of his illness and what lies ahead may, right to his death, speak with his family as though he is as ignorant of it all, as they had hoped and indeed worked for him to be.

I learned much from an occasion when a patient asked to speak to me and proceeded to go through a check list of 22 questions ranging from how he would die to possible hymns for his funeral service! Suddenly, his wife's face appeared round his bedside curtains and, quick as a flash, his face broke into a smile as he said 'Oh darling, I wish you could have been here. Doctor has just been discussing cars with me and suggests that for our touring holiday in Spain next year we would be better with a new Metro!' Later the wife demanded to see me to upbraid me for daring to suggest that her husband (who died five days later) had any idea of how ill he was. Their mutual behaviour towards each other was, however, quite appropriate. He showed his love by protecting her, and his pragmatism by discussing every question that mattered to him with someone who could bear to help him. *She* was happy to think that she had shielded him as she must have done so often in their life together.

At other times, the growth of a human spirit approaching death may mystify relatives, or even hurt them, and here the doctor has a special role. Often the selfish man becomes unexpectedly considerate and generous; the shy person becomes more outgoing and confident; the critical or abrasive one becomes appreciative and gentle. This is not the effect of psychotropic drugs or the result of cerebral metastases, but the response of the human spirit that comes when someone is nursed in an atmosphere of love and support, free from bitterness, aggression, conflict, and destructive criticism. After a lifetime of domestic strife and mutual resentment this 'new person' image can be particularly hurtful for the one who is being left behind. 'How can he be so charming now after the way he has treated me for 30 years?'

PROTECTING THE RELATIVES

This leads us to look at another aspect of caring for the dying—caring for their relatives. A general practitioner will not need to be reminded that the immediate relatives are as much his concern as the patient is. Indeed, he may look forward to being their trusted doctor and friend for many years to come. In hospital, all attention seems to be focused on the patient, and hospital doctors tend to pay less attention to the needs of relatives than they merit, judging by studies carried out in a number of centres.

The needs of relatives are obviously different from those of the patient and may be skilfully concealed behind questions that seem to be entirely about the patient and his welfare. Through experience, it becomes clearer that much of their concern about the patient's suffering is not only a reflection of their love but also of their guilt (unjustified as it may be), their sense of failure or inadequacy, and their profound (and often quite justified) apprehension about their own future.

CARING FOR RELATIVES

The doctor who confines himself to speaking to relatives only about the patient, his investigations, treatment, prognosis, etc., and fails to ask '. . . and now tell me how *you* are getting on' is failing to understand the breadth of his professional role. A patient's improved appetite in hospital may be seen as an indication of his wife's culinary inadequacy at home. His relaxed mood may be construed as the result of his being taken out of her anxious care, or his persisting pain and discomfort as due to her nursing incompetence.

Similar examples abound. For the patient, death is the end of suffering, possibly (if he is blessed with a faith) the promise of better things to come. For the relative, death is only the beginning of a chapter of life so different, so daunting, that he or she can scarcely bear to look into the future.

Nothing could be more important for patient or relative (for their delicately interwoven reactions influence symptoms and prognosis) than for the doctor *always* to set time aside for the *personal, particular* needs of the relatives. The one who is to be left must be invited and encouraged to express how he or she really feels. To the doctor's surprise, a wife may describe how relieved she is to know that her husband's death is imminent because that will signal the end of his suffering *or* the chance for her of a new life that can only be better than the one she has endured for many years. She may just want to say how uncomfortable it is to sit by the bedside or how upsetting it is to see him so changed for better or worse. She may want to be reassured that someone will visit and support her after the death during the months and years that will bring loneliness and a sense of 'aloneness' she has never known before. While the patient may regain a faith, so the relatives may lose faith and find it replaced with bitterness and anger, often directed at the medical profession or even God himself. Relatives, every bit as much as patients, need to be given encouragement and permission to 'be themselves', to express their true feelings, whether tearful, angry, relieved, or fearful, and to be accepted as they are.

A widow once remarked to me that she wished I could be as good with relatives as I had been with the patient, her late husband. 'I used to feel so angry with you when you came downstairs each day, put an arm on my shoulder, and told me how well I was caring for him. You never once asked me how I really felt, about how angry I was, how frightened, how let down!' Such conversations with relatives about their personal feelings must, obviously, be confidential, but this need not prevent the doctor telling the patient that he is meeting with the relatives to try to help them too, provided that at all times he reassures the patient that there are no secrets being withheld from him.

At the heart of all 'talking with the dying' must be complete honesty and openness, founded on professional skill, competence, and empathy. Only a foolish doctor believes he must appear omnipotent! His patients, and particularly those who are dying and their families, are likely to recognize his frailties, but usually respect him all the more for them if, in every single encounter, he remains a friend who can express humanity, humility, and humour.

14 Talking about sexual function

The need for doctors to desexualize the intimacy of clinical work has been identified in earlier chapters as a factor that inhibits them from discussing patients' sexual function, or even other 'personal' matters. Nevertheless, with insight and training this reluctance can and should be overcome, since problems of sexual function are not rarities. Surveys in general practice have shown that 10–15 per cent of patients have a sexual problem of some sort.

However, enquiries about a patient's sexual function should not form a regular part of routine history-taking. First, the doctor has to consider carefully the nature of the patient's presenting symptoms, their possible causes, and likely consequences. Enquiry would certainly be appropriate when a patient's physical condition or current medication could affect normal sexual function, or when the presenting complaint is vague ('feeling run down', 'being out of sorts', 'not feeling my normal self'), without obvious explanation, or when there are indications of unexplained anxiety or depression.

As in other areas of medicine, it is helpful to keep in mind the epidemiology of the disorder i.e. the circumstances in which the prevalence of sexual difficulty is likely to be greater and when, therefore, enquiry would be appropriate. These include situations such as

- the patient first seeking contraceptive advice;
- the patient presenting with symptoms of possible sexually-transmitted disease;
- the woman presenting with her first pregnancy;
- the woman appearing for postnatal examination;
- the patient who has undergone surgical mutilation, e.g. mastectomy, a bowel stoma, an amputation;
- the woman with a gynaecological complaint, particularly one causing genital pain or tenderness;

- the patient with a disorder likely to result in sexual dysfunction, e.g. diabetes, alcohol abuse, multiple sclerosis, severe arthritis;
- the patient receiving medication that can affect sexual function, e.g. some hypotensive drugs, psychotropics, diuretics;
- the patient, male or female, experiencing climacteric symptoms;
- the patient who indicates that there are problems in the marital relationship.

HOW TO INTRODUCE THE TOPIC

Broaching the topic of sexual function during history-taking calls for delicacy combined with directness. Timing is important, and rapport with the patient should first be established. The questions asked should be unambiguous, and should convey by their openness the doctor's comfort with the topic and readiness to talk. The vocabulary chosen should consist of words that the patient is likely to understand, not too formally 'medical', nor slangy or vulgar.

The pattern of enquiry depends on whether the patient has acknowledged the existence of a sexual problem, or whether the doctor has decided to take the initiative in raising the topic because he believes it to be relevant to the patient's complaints. Considering the latter situation first: if the patient is married, a suitable simple direct question would be 'Are you able to enjoy sexual intercourse comfortably?' In the case of an older person, the question could be modified 'Are you still able to enjoy sexual intercourse comfortably?' If the patient answers affirmatively to such an enquiry, usually no more questions need be asked. Questions in these terms do not imply that a sexual problem exists, and are therefore likely to be received better than the enquiry 'Do you have a sexual problem?'

When the patient is single and the doctor does not know whether a sexual relationship exists or not, it may appear best to enquire about boyfriends or girlfriends before asking 'Are you having a sexual relationship?' Alternatively, and perhaps preferably, a simple direct approach can again be adopted. A useful question from which to begin, particularly with a young teenager, would be 'Have you ever had sexual intercourse?' This takes account of the tentative and sporadic nature of much sexual activity in the teenage years. If the answer is 'Yes', then 'Have you a partner now?' is appropriate, followed by the same sort of question described for a married person, 'Are you able to enjoy sexual intercourse comfortably?'

When the patient is ostensibly without a partner—divorced, widowed, or separated—particular tact is required. In the case of a widow or widower, the doctor may prefer first to ask tentatively 'How do you cope with your sexual feelings since you lost your partner?' But again it may be more fitting to ask directly 'Have you met a new sexual partner since you were divorced/separated/widowed?'

Turning to the situation in which the patient has indicated that a sexual problem exists, sometimes the complaint is vague or unspecified 'Well, to be honest, doctor, I want to talk to you about my sex life. It's a disaster area!' 'Actually, doctor, I've lost all interest in married life.' 'I guess I'm not much use to my wife nowadays.' It can then be helpful to explore the difficulty initially with one or two more general questions about the patient's subjective experience, such as

'Do you look forward to making love?'
'Do you get aroused/turned on?'
'Does love-making make you feel happy and relaxed?'
'Do you find intercourse uncomfortable or painful?'

Questions of this sort, in opening up the topic, allow patients to talk first about their general sexual feelings and responses. Then it is appropriate to find out what specific difficulties occur. If the patient has not already given an indication of what is going wrong, the questions should cover the main aspects of sexual response. For a woman, does good lubrication occur with arousal, Does she get wet enough? Is satisfaction (climax) usually attained? For a man, is there difficulty in getting or keeping an erection? Does the man come (ejaculate) too quickly?

Once a clearer picture of the difficulties has been obtained, the doctor should find out when and how the problem started. It is often useful to go back to the start of the relationship. Was there difficulty then, and if not, when did the problem develop? Were there any concurrent events that might have led to the problem, e.g. illness, loss of a job, strain in the relationship, infidelity, bereavement? It is usually appropriate to ask at some point in the history how often the couple make love and, if intercourse is infrequent, when the last time was. More general questions are then called for about the couple's opportunities for affectionate interaction. Do they go out and about much together? Do they display affection outside the bedroom? Do they usually go to bed together? Who usually makes the first move? Does the couple share any physical affection that is not just a preliminary to coitus?

When sexual unresponsiveness is part of the problem, the patient can be asked whether feelings of sexual interest occur when the partner is not present or when intercourse is not in prospect.

To have a better understanding of the patient's current difficulties, it is often helpful to discover more about attitudes to sexuality acquired during childhood, and about the earliest sexual experiences:

• What sex education did the patient receive as a child?

• Were sexual matters something that could be discussed in the home?

• What warnings or prohibitions did the patient receive as a child?

• Was the patient as a child fondled or otherwise sexually exploited by an adult, particularly a member of the family?

• Did any sexually alarming episodes occur during childhood or adolescence?

Regarding early sexual experience, it might be seen as accusatory to ask 'Was your husband/wife/fiancé(e) the first person you ever made love to?' A better question is 'Can you remember your very first sexual experience? When did that happen?' From this beginning it will be possible to trace the patient's sexual relationship(s), and to discover whether difficulties similar to the current ones were present earlier.

If the doctor has had no special training or experience in helping patients with sexual problems, he may feel that, having identified the problem, the best course is to refer the patient to someone with appropriate skills. If, however, he decides to find out more about the problem, the sort of information required can be summarized under the following headings.

Erectile impotence

Erectile impotence can be due to organic or functional causes, and appropriate questions should provide a pointer. Do normal erections occur on waking from dreaming sleep, and during fantasy and masturbation? If the impotence is limited to situations where intercourse is attempted or is in prospect, is an erection achieved and then lost, or is there complete erectile failure? When the condition is secondary (i.e. preceded by normal erectile function), it is important to know whether the onset was gradual or abrupt.

Premature ejaculation

Establish whether ejaculation is controlled more easily during masturbation. After ejaculating once, can the man become aroused again and continue for longer before ejaculating on the second occasion?

Failure to ejaculate

These cases are by no means rare, and may present as unexplained infertility. One should find out whether the difficulty is situational, i.e. whether it is only within the vagina that the patient has difficulty in ejaculating. Is there a history of practising coitus interruptus or reservatus during early sexual experience?

In female patients, the commonest problem is some form of *sexual unresponsiveness*, usually secondary. It is important to distinguish between lack of sexual interest or appetite (the woman who never thinks or feels 'sexy'); impaired responsiveness (the woman who feels interest, but fails to respond during love-making); and orgasmic difficulty (failure to climax). It is helpful to enquire whether the patient is more responsive to manual caresses than to vaginal coitus. Can she experience arousal by masturbating? Do her difficulties relate only to her present partner? Does her partner spend enough time in foreplay? Is he rough, indifferent, or demanding? Does he ejaculate too quickly?

Vaginismus

These cases are likely to present as failure to consummate a marriage (sometimes after many years) or as unexplained infertility. Can the patient allow anything to enter her vagina? Her own finger? Her partner's finger? A tampon? Did she experience alarming episodes or admonitions in childhood? Can she experience satisfactory arousal if penetration is not attempted?

Most patients with sexual problems are quite ready to talk about them to a doctor who shows concern, understanding, and, perhaps most importantly, comfort with the topic. As the doctor learns the appropriate way to phrase his questions, he will be surprised to discover how easy it is to include this important aspect of health in his history-taking.

15 Aspects of transcultural communication

With travellers, visitors, and immigrants from many countries of the world now very much part of the everyday scene, doctors need to broaden their understanding of how best to communicate with patients from other cultures, avoiding the difficulties that can arise through ignorance of the customs and beliefs of other communities.

LANGUAGE

If patient and doctor do not have a common language, they may have to communicate through an interpreter. A relative, a trusted friend, or even a stranger of the same sex as the patient can fulfil this role. Sometimes a teenage child of the family who has been educated in Britain may be the person in the family with the best command of English. Many hospitals have a panel of volunteer interpreters covering a wide range of languages. Vocabulary, nevertheless, can present problems. There may be lack of appropriate corresponding words to describe both physical and emotional symptoms, and changes of mood.

Even during interviews with native English-speaking patients, terms used either by the patient or by the doctor may be confusing and ambiguous and readily give rise to serious misconceptions.

Examples of this sort of difficulty (from the field of neurology) were given by Hawkes [66]. Terms such as weakness, numbness, giddy or dizzy turns, neuritis, or migraine, for example, are liable to be used by doctors and patients without a clear mutual understanding of what the term is supposed to mean. These difficulties are much more likely to arise when the patient is from a different culture and speaks a different language.

Besides this, the patient's perception of his complaint and interpretation of the nature of his illness are likely to be much influenced by cultural frames of reference. For example, feeling unwell may be construed as a consequence of such diverse influences as astrological fate, impiety, a curse or spell, or even 'possession' by a spirit. These varying notions have a profound influence on the manner in which the complaint is described. A full review of culture-bound syndromes of illness-behaviour has been prepared by Littlewood and Lipsedge [67].

INFLUENCE OF FAMILY STRUCTURE AND RELATIONSHIPS

Among the strongest elements of cultural influence are those bound up with the pattern of everyday family living. In many traditional cultures, particularly in rural settings, the family is a compound group of members, with several generations living together, and with young wives joining the family on marriage.

The head of the family

In most of these traditional cultures, the senior male is regarded as very much the head of the family, whatever the influence the older women customarily exercise backstage, in the privacy of the domestic circle! The approval of the male head of the family may therefore be considered necessary not only for major interventions such as an operation, but for any decision about the medical care of any member of the family. Further, it may be helpful when a consultation takes place to involve the head of the family whenever possible in the exposition, since compliance is likely to depend crucially on his endorsement and reiteration of the doctor's instructions.

The roles and attitudes of women

Where traditional cultures are still strong, the social roles of women are very much centred in the domestic world—home-making, the preparation of food, child-bearing and child-rearing. In rural communities, these functions are often combined with many of the most laborious family tasks, such as growing food, carrying water, and gathering fuel.

In Islamic cultures, women may be expected to seclude themselves in the harem (*zenana*), the women's quarters of the home. When they venture outside the home, 'respectable' women avoid social (and certainly physical) contact with strangers. In orthodox Hindu communities, also, women seek, wherever possible, to avoid contact with others, particularly those of a lower caste.

These cultural patterns and attitudes exercise an important influence on many aspects of the lives of the women concerned. Females are likely to have received fewer years of schooling, to be less literate and less able to speak English, so that verbal and written communication can be much more difficult. Women, therefore, usually seek advice and information about aspects of their personal lives, including health matters, from older women, generally within the family, rather than from books, magazines, the media, and professional sources. Conversely, those women who do find themselves 'isolated' in a nuclear family may feel insecure, unsupported, and less able to make decisions for themselves.

A married woman's social standing is mainly derived from her reputation for 'respectability', i.e. conformity to the conventions of the culture, from the number of her children (particularly her sons), and from her seniority within the family group.

An unmarried female's good standing in southern Asian cultures is crucially dependent on her reputation for chaste behaviour—the assurance of her virginity. Women's need to protect their personal reputations throughout their lives has an influence not only on their general social behaviour but also on their attitudes towards clinical examination, with the undressing and exposure that inevitably occurs. A Hindu woman might cover her face with the hem of her sari during abdominal palpation, and is likely to adopt an expression of rather exaggerated distaste during vaginal examination, to emphasize her respectability and her aversion to the intimate contact with a man other than her husband. Many traditional women agree to clinical examination only if it is performed by a female doctor.

The exclusiveness and privacy that characterize a couple's physical relationship in marriage make it difficult for either of them to discuss this aspect of their lives, even with a doctor of the same sex. In an arranged marriage, the wife, in particular, may have quite modest expectations of sexual fulfilment, and she is for that reason less likely to sense that a sexual problem exists; and even if she does, she may well not think it seemly for a wife to voice such concerns.

The compound family

Relationships within the compound family are generally dominated by the hierarchy of age, the younger members regularly deferring to their elders. Even a small difference of age between siblings implies a corresponding ranking, and an obligation to defer. The senior, older members of the family almost automatically attract respect and prestige; their increasing dependence and their idiosyncracies are accepted; and the responsibility for their care is usually shouldered without hesitation. Indeed, the proposal that an elderly relative be removed to hospital may be construed as a reflection upon the caring of the other family members, and therefore resisted. This exemplifies the sense of collective responsibility and mutual obligation within the compound family, even when all the members do not live under the same roof. Important decisions are made only after consultation within the family group.

The corollary of the respect accorded to the elderly is the submission and conformity expected of the young, and of the adolescent in particular. If this is not forthcoming, as is more likely to happen in an established immigrant family whose children have received all their education in Britain, great tension or even serious rifts can arise between the generations. These may centre on disagreements about conventional dressing, about choice of friends, or about social mixing with the opposite sex, but become more serious when the parents are planning an arranged marriage for their son or daughter who wishes to find his or her own partner.

Children

Throughout history, children have been seen as a family's great asset, a blessing from God. In communities dependent on peasant agriculture, children's contribution to the labour force is invaluable, especially during labour-intensive periods such as harvest. Sons in particular endow the family with greater financial security, with physical security (for the women, the land, the home) and with social security as the parents grow older. In Hindu culture, a son also affords spiritual security, through his important role in the funeral rites of his parents.

But, for countless generations past, families have experienced the relentless toll of heavy infant and child mortality. Commonly, a half or more of those born have failed to survive to reach adolescence. A woman might expect only two surviving sons after bearing seven or eight children. As a consequence, in traditional cultures, pregnancy is celebrated, and children are welcomed, cossetted, and spoiled by their grandparents. Large families are idealized. Fertility is greatly valued, and infertility is regarded as the ultimate disaster.

High maternal mortality has also been an 'accepted' part of human experience from earliest times, and in many parts of the world high maternal mortality persists [68]. In those communities in which maternal mortality was high and fertility was uncontrolled, the life expectancy of women was strikingly *less* than that of men, in contrast to the longevity of women in the contemporary developed world. This experience must also have played an important part in shaping cultural attitudes to favour early marriage and high fertility. Unless a woman married early and bred frequently throughout her short life, the family might be in danger of extinction.

These deep-seated cultural values often engender suspicion and hostility towards the control of fertility: towards contraception, sterilization, or abortion. Similarly, women refuse to consider hysterectomy, however severe their gynaecological problems. It is only when the survival of children can be demonstrated and assured that couples become willing to discuss contraception, and to contemplate restricting the size of their family.

The precarious nature of a young child's hold on life is acknowledged in a number of customs in different communities. The infant's hair may not be cut for many months, to avoid weakening it in any way. In the Indian tradition, dark powder (*kohl, surma*) is applied round the child's eyes, to 'protect' the child from illness. This powder sometimes contains lead compounds, which may poison the child. In some cultures, the child's naming ceremony is deferred for some considerable time after its birth to conceal, as it were, the child's existence and identity from malevolent influences. In the Arab tradition, a child should not be admired, nor should complimentary comments be made about its good looks or good health, lest some harm comes upon the child through the 'evil eye'.

RELIGIOUS BELIEFS AND PRACTICES

Bodily cleanliness is regarded in many cultures as a religious duty, and therefore in some sense a mark of piety. 'Cleanliness is next to godliness.' Hindus aim to bathe each morning in flowing water (not a stagnant bath!). They wash the anal region with water after defaecation, and generally regard a menstruating woman as ritually' unclean, so that in some traditions she may not even enter the kitchen to prepare food. The faeces or other bodily secretions of another person, particularly one of low caste, are considered highly 'unclean', polluting those who come in contact with them. Muslims, too, consider bodily cleanliness a virtue, and wash ritually before each of their daily prayer times. Muslim women take a ritual bath at the end of each menstrual period, after which they are able to resume intercourse. If asked the date of their last menstrual period these patients give the date of the *last*, not the first, day.

These attitudes to cleanliness and pollution may make it very difficult for a patient to accept the idea of a bowel stoma, and faecal or urinary incontinence can create great distress, making the patient feel a virtual outcast. Because nurses have to deal with excreta, nursing may be seen as a degrading low-status occupation, and nurses may be accorded less respect for this reason.

Food and fasting play an important part in the religious life of many cultures. A Muslim will not partake of pork, and will eat other meat only if the animal was ritually slaughtered (*halal* meat). An orthodox Jew does not eat dairy products and meat at the same meal, and again his meat must be correctly slaughtered (*kosher*). Many Hindus are exclusively vegetarian and those who are not would generally not eat beef or pork. During the lunar month of Ramadan, devout Muslims fast between sunrise and sunset. Hindus may fast on particular holy days each week or month.

These dietary observances can create great difficulty for the patient in hospital, who may refuse much of the food that is offered to him, and may prefer to eat only the food brought in by his relatives. Apart from these more stringent observances, dietary choice may be restricted by other beliefs about food. In Indian culture it is generally held that some foods (vegetable oil, maize or millet flour, unrefined sugar, strong spices, onions) are 'hot', and therefore stimulating or even aphrodisiac, whereas others (milk, butter, wheat flour, rice, white sugar, honey) are 'cool', and so are safer and less disturbing. If sexual restraint (or even asceticism) is deemed a religious virtue and a prerequisite for good health, certain 'hot' foods may have to be avoided altogether.

In this context, it is important also to understand how loss of semen, whether from nocturnal emission, spermatorrhoea, masturbation, or frequent coitus, has become in some Asian cultures a common source of sustained anxiety among males. In the ancient tradition of the Vedas, semen was considered to be a sort of vital essence, a source of psychic energy and well-being. It was said to be formed from blood, each drop of semen requiring forty drops of blood and forty days for its 'distillation'. As a legacy of these beliefs in some cultures, normal fatigue or impaired concentration may be construed as symptoms of depletion of semen, and anxious men may become obsessionally concerned about seminal loss.

ATTITUDES TO OBESITY

In areas of the world where most people are too poor to be able to afford a nourishing diet, and the really poor are evidently underweight because of inadequate nutrition, obesity naturally becomes a cultural mark of affluence and social status, something to be proud of in one's self, one's spouse, and one's children. In this setting, advice to reduce weight is likely to be ignored.

ATTITUDES TO LIFE EVENTS: FATE AND DEATH

Most religions acknowledge the influence of a supernatural force or forces in the affairs of humankind. Devout believers, whether Christians, Muslims, or Hindus, feel their fate is in the hands of a higher being. Just as Christians may qualify their future plans with 'd.v.' (*deo volente*), so Muslims, in speaking of future events, add '*ensh-Allah*' (if God wills), the same qualifying words. In Hindu culture, trust in astrology and horoscopes is strong, and behind this is belief in the recurring cycle of reincarnation, in the course of which the soul is inexorably requited or rewarded for behaviour in a previous life (*karma*).

All these various influences tend to create an underlying feeling that a person's fate or destiny is pre-ordained, and that a wise man accepts his powerlessness to control or even influence events in his own life. Such fatalism can make easier the acceptance of suffering, death, bereavement, or disability, but is also liable to engender a passivity towards events and to weaken any readiness to strive, overcome, or wrestle with the 'foul clutch of circumstance'.

The acceptance of death is not only a matter of fatalism. Death in the traditional cultures of the Third World is also accepted more. readily because it is a common event in the past experience of the family, especially the death of children, and also because ready access to life-saving medical care is not the normal expectation.

The rituals of death and mourning among different religious faiths were well described by Black [43]. The head of a dying Muslim should be turned towards Mecca by moving the bed. As soon as possible after death, the members of a Muslim family will wish to take the body, so that it can be ritually washed by Muslim hands, with prayers, and so prepared for burial, wrapped in a clean white sheet, on the same day if possible. Both Muslims and Hindus (but not Sikhs) hold that only fellow-believers should touch the dead body; others should wear gloves. After abortion, a Muslim couple will usually wish to treat the body of the fetus with similar respect, before burial.

Hindus often prefer to die at home, accompanied by prayers. The body is again washed ritually by family members, and so prepared for cremation. However, still births and children under the age of about four years are not usually cremated, but buried. The eldest son's participation in the funeral rituals (whenever possible) is believed to be necessary for the true rest of the departed soul. After cremation, the ashes (in Britain) may be scattered over any large expanse of water. There is a prescribed period of 12 days mourning, during which white clothes are worn.

Where death occurs, Muslims and orthodox Jews oppose post-mortem examination, and in other cultures too there is reluctance to allow the body of a dead relative to be mutilated in this way. For similar reasons, donation of organs such as kidneys may be quite unacceptable, except possibly for the benefit of a close relative. While the loyalties within the compound family are very strong, they can also be somewhat insular. As a result, the sense of social obligation to give blood (for example) may be limited to the family, or the clan or caste group.

HEALTH BELIEFS AND PRACTICES

Every community has a varied store of traditional homely remedies, especially for common ailments. In many cultures, a more formal system of traditional medicine exists, and the practitioners may have acquired their knowledge and skills through apprenticeship or by more systematic instruction. The ancient systems of Chinese and Indian (Ayurvedic) medicine rely heavily on herbal preparations, but also utilize exotic remedies prepared from animal products, precious stones, or metals, for example. African traditional medicine encompasses a wide range of practitioners, including bonesetters, surgeons, and manipulators, as well as spirit-healers. Exorcism has been seen as an occasional remedy in Britain and other countries for many centuries past.

In Chinese traditional therapeutics, acupuncture plays an important part. Just as Roman Catholics might wear St Christopher medallions, and fundamentalist Protestants have their promise boxes packed with reassuring Biblical verses, in Islamic communities amulets containing verses from the Koran are commonly worn as a protection from illness, and traditional therapy may include a potion prepared by washing a Koranic verse from a slate. Moxibustion, cupping, bleeding, and cauterization are other methods of traditional therapy.

Much nearer home, what are generally known as 'alternative therapies' (see the BMA report [69]) have become fashionable in recent years. These include osteopathy, chiropractic, homoeopathy, herbalism, massage, aroma and foot therapy, yoga, and faith healing. Even in a culture in which scientific medicine holds strong sway over people's minds and outlooks, some individuals seek health or healing through unusual modalities of treatment, in some cases based on quite bizarre beliefs.

Sometimes patients from a traditional culture may feel it wise to aim for the best of both worlds, and so consult an orthodox practitioner while concurrently seeking the advice of a traditional healer, or taking a traditional remedy on their own initiative. Some of these patients from other cultures who prefer western medicine show reluctance to place full trust in the opinion of a single doctor. They may consult independently two or three doctors, or even more if they have the means, as if the best advice would emerge from a sort of ballot of medical opinion. Their behaviour, if brought into the open, is likely to antagonize the doctors concerned, because of the implied lack of confidence.

What appears to be distrust of doctors can sometimes be shown by American patients, because of the manner in which they are liable to interrogate the doctor over seeming minutiae, may expect laboratory tests to validate the diagnosis, and demand something more than the usual explanation for each step in management. Often this appearance of distrust is little more than a desire for greater and more informed involvement in matters concerning the individual's health, but it may be intensified because of the commercialism of some American practice.

This short chapter provides no more than a few illustrative glimpses of various cultural patterns and practices, and of the way in which these can affect communication between patient and doctor. Empathy, on which good communication so vitally depends, presents the doctor with a much more difficult challenge when cultural boundaries have to be crossed.

16 Developing the skills

Central to the theme of this book is the conviction that skill in interviewing is principally a product of professional learning, rather than an innate ability that some are born with and some are born without. It is sometimes claimed that students should be selected for admission to medical schools partly on the basis of their ability to communicate, that only 'outgoing' personalities should be accepted, in the hope that all doctors would, almost automatically, turn out to be good communicators. Perhaps some form of personality and aptitude testing might be a fruitful part of the selection process, rather than reliance solely on the student's ability to score well in a narrow range of science subjects in school qualifying exams. However, given the range of careers a medical graduate may pursue—in clinical, administrative, laboratory, investigative, or military medicine, for example—it would be difficult to specify the particular qualities to be required in every entrant.

UNFAVOURABLE INFLUENCES

There is some evidence that the process of undergraduate medical education may, in some instances, inhibit rather than promote the development of interviewing skills. One or two studies have shown this effect [70,71], which might be a consequence of the traditional pre-clinical/clinical divide in the medical curriculum. If a student is 'imprinted' with a conceptual framework of function and disease based solely on the physical sciences, he may acquire a view of patients as disordered machines before he even begins to learn to talk to them as people.

There is no doubt that early and continuing contact with patients is important in promoting the facility for good communication. But when the student does start regular clinical work in the wards,

Fig. 16.1 The ward round: an example of poor communication

he may be presented with a poor model of doctor–patient communication during traditional ward rounds. As the hierarchical
retinue of doctors, students, and nurses processes around the ward,
communication with patients may well be overshadowed by the
intra-professional exchanges at the foot of the bed, since the
medical staff are, it has to be admitted, often preoccupied with a
professionally centred game of one-up-manship, which Arluke has
called 'roundsmanship' [72] (Fig. 16.1).

The pitfalls and obstacles that can stand in the way of good
communication during ward rounds have been well described by
Steele and Morton [73]. They include lack of privacy, inadequate
explanation, and open criticism of staff or students, as well as
behaviour such as ignoring or excluding the patient, and 'exhibit-
ing' the patient.

ACTIVE DEVELOPMENT OF INTERVIEWING SKILLS

Students can best develop their skill in interviewing by participating in or observing, and then discussing, actual interviews. This learning process is most fruitful when conducted in a small group of (say) six to ten students with a tutor. The opportunities for detailed learning are greatly enhanced if the interviews can be recorded on videotape (or even audio tape) so that, with play-back, precise recall and review of the exchanges during each interview are possible. Video methods, of course, also allow the non-verbal elements in the interaction between doctor and patient to be studied carefully [74].

When this format of learning is being used, one of the students takes the part of the doctor, while the 'patient' may be a real patient who has consented to participate. Many patients are happy to assist in this way if the purpose of the exercise is carefully explained to them, because of their awareness of the importance of improving doctors' communication skills. Alternatively, a simulated patient can be used. This individual may be a medical teacher or a lay volunteer (possibly an amateur actor) who has been briefed to play a particular patient role.

However, the best opportunities for new learning during this type of exercise occur when a second student plays the role of the patient, guided by a written advance brief. The student entering into the part of a patient has to reflect on how that patient would feel and behave in a particular situation, and so his capacity for empathy develops and his learning can be shared with other students in the group [75].

Other advantages of using a role-played patient are that the real patients are not inconvenienced and the tutor can freely choose the clinical problem on which the group will centre, rather than being confined to the range of clinical cases present within the ward or clinic on that particular day.

FURTHER LEARNING

We have reviewed the skills of affective communication in the general context of everyday consultations with a variety of patients.

There are additional specific skills that need to be used in particular situations, for instance with blind patients, deaf or aphasic patients, or those who can be spoken to only through an interpreter. In other sections of the book, the special problems of affective communication that arise in caring for dying patients, or in helping the patient with sexual difficulties, have been emphasized. Again, specific skills are called for in these situations. There is always more to learn!

I have deliberately not sought to explore those dimensions of dialogue that are generally referred to as 'counselling', in which an important aim is to assist the client/patient to resolve for himself difficulties in his relationships with others, and in the process to reach a greater degree of self-understanding and self-reliance. Similarly, I have not called upon the interpretive constructs of the doctor–patient relationship derived from depth psychology (psychoanalysis), as expounded by Balint and his school [76]. In pursuing this analytical approach, the doctor has to be ready to submit his own attitudes and feelings to open self- and peer-group scrutiny.

Not all doctors have the time, inclination, or aptitude to adopt these models of patient–doctor interaction. I have attempted to outline a less sophisticated approach, appropriate for everyday use, and to identify certain inhibitory influences that must be recognized and overcome. It is my hope that an understanding of these factors will promote improved interviewing skills and the adoption of a more sensitive and empathic clinical style. In consequence, tomorrow's medical graduates may be less likely to evoke from their patients the sorts of justifiable criticism that were discussed at the outset. At the same time, they will enhance their clinical problem-solving skills in line with the need so clearly spelled out in the report 'Physicians for the Twentyfirst Century' [77].

Résumé

The purpose of this book has been to demonstrate that effective, sensitive communication calls for specific skills, which can be defined through analysis of actual interviews and developed through understanding and practice. It is a fallacy to rely on just being one's self—on being 'natural'. In fact, the spontaneous human feelings that are liable to be evoked during interviews with patients, whether feelings of sympathy or aversion, attraction or repulsion, have to be controlled and modified by the doctor's professionalism.

When these professional skills are well deployed, the effect is not to isolate the doctor from the patient. On the contrary, a clinical setting is created within which the doctor feels secure enough to reduce the distance between himself and the patient while retaining an appropriate degree of professional detachment. At the same time, the patient is helped to voice feelings and concerns that might otherwise have remained unexpressed.

Detachment and involvement are both, in a measure, necessary attributes of the professional's role. But it is fair to say that doctors generally, in seeking a balance between them, have inclined traditionally towards detachment. Maintaining a greater distance from the patient can appear very attractive. It reinforces the doctor's authority; it insulates a doctor from the patient's distress; it helps to dissociate the doctor from any possible sense of failure. Involvement, in contrast, can seem rather threatening and burdensome. It might put pressure on the doctor beyond his capacity; it might create discomfort in coping with emotions; it could eventually culminate in 'burn-out' if the doctor allowed his involvement to become too intense or too prolonged.

I have endeavoured in this volume to outline a professional attitude and manner that avoids either extreme, and which therefore has, I believe, a better claim to the epithet 'professional'. It aims to meet the expectation voiced by many patients at the present time that their doctors should not just be competent diagnosticians and good technicians (however important that may be) but should also bring to their work the skills and attitudes of caring. This implies, above all, the sort of sensitive and open inter-personal communication that I have sought to describe.

Appendix

This outline is based on guidance notes given to medical students at the University of Edinburgh, under the auspices of the Medical Education Committee.

First, list the patient's *presenting complaints*, as far as possible in his own words. Give a brief chronological narrative of their onset. It may be necessary to interview a third party in the case of children; confused, inebriated, or unconscious patients; and those suffering from severe emotional disorders or mental illness.

The *characteristics of each symptom* should be defined in some detail:

- duration;
- mode of onset—sudden or gradual;
- possible association, e.g. exercise, meals, movement, emotional tension;
- periodicity—nocturnal pattern, interference with sleep;
- progression;
- localization;
- premonitory, precipitating, aggravating, or relieving factors;
- effect on patient's everyday life.

Past medical history

Previous illnesses, operations and other health problems should be listed, with a note of the date or patient's age at the time. Remember that inaccuracies and omissions are common.

Note any hypersensitivity to drugs, X-ray contrast media, or other agents.

Drug history

Identify all current medication, and all treatment previously given for the present illness. Was it effective? Were there any abnormal reactions?

Alcohol consumption should be estimated quantitatively. What is the pattern of drinking? Is there evidence of dependence?

Smoking: present and past habits. Is there any other 'social' drug use?

Obstetric history (females)

State the total number of pregnancies and abortions. Note complications of pregnancy or labour. Enquire about the current health of any children. Note the method(s) of contraception used, if any.

Comprehensive enquiry: check-list of symptoms

Symptoms not present can be recorded thus: dyspnoea—0.

General

Weight loss or gain, energy, sleep pattern, general well-being—if vague, enquire 'When did you last feel well?'

Cardiovascular system

- Dyspnoea
- Ankle oedema
- Chest pain—on exertion or at rest
- Palpitations
- Intermittent claudication

Respiratory system

- Cough; sputum (colour, amount)
- Dyspnoea; wheeze
- Haemoptysis
- Chest pain

Gastro-intestinal system

- Appetite; dietary pattern
- Weight change
- Dysphagia

- Indigestion; heartburn; waterbrash
- Nausea; vomiting
- Abdominal pain—continuous/colicky
- Bowel habit—recent change; stools—blood/pallor/odour/ mucus/incontinence
- Jaundice

Renal and genito-urinary system

- Thirst
- Micturition—frequency; polyuria; nocturia
- Dysuria; hesitancy; impaired stream; urgency
- Incontinence—stress/urge/complete
- Haematuria; urine colour/frothiness
- Lumbar or loin pain
- Balanitis; urethral discharge
- Sexual function
    In men—impotence; premature ejaculation
    In women—dyspareunia; impaired desire or response
- (Women) Menstrual function
    Age of menarche; cycle length; duration and amount of menstrual flow
    Date of last period
    If no longer menstruating, date of menopause; any post-menopausal bleeding
    Leukorrhoea; pruritus vulvae

Central nervous system

- Impaired vision—acuity/field of vision/diplopia
- Impaired hearing; tinnitus
- Fainting/fits/black-outs/dizziness/vertigo
- Headaches; loss of consciousness
- Loss of sensation; paraesthesiae
- Paralysis; paresis
- Mood impairment; sleep pattern; early-morning waking

Skin

- Itching (pruritus)
- Rashes; eruptions—petechiae—bruising
- Contact with plants, pets, etc.

Locomotor system
- Impaired mobility
- Difficulty in walking—limp/unsteadiness/loss of balance
- Backache
- Joint pain or swelling
- Muscle pain—cramps—weakness
- Postures that relieve or aggravate the pain
- Use of sticks or other aids

Family history

Review all first-degree relatives (parents, children, siblings). Record present age and state of health. If dead, state cause, and reactions to bereavement in the family. Note occurrence of similar or associated diseases within the family.

Social history

This should encompass the following.
- the patient's household circumstances and occupational environment;
- some impression of the patient's lifestyle;
- inter-personal relationships at home and at work;
- occupational history—employed/unemployed; stability of job tenure; occupational hazards;
- travel abroad—alone/with partner; countries visited.

References

1. Nuffield Provincial Hospitals Trust (1980). *Talking with patients: a teaching approach*. Oxford University Press, Oxford.
2. Stiles, W.B. *et al.* (1979). Interaction exchange structure and patient satisfaction with medical interviews. *Medical Care*, **17**, 667–81.
3. Comstock, L.M. *et al.* (1982). Physician behaviours that correlate with patient satisfaction. *Journal of Medical Education*, **57**, 105–12.
4. Korsch, B.M., Gozzi, E.K., and Francis, V. (1968). Doctor–patient interaction and patient satisfaction. *Paediatrics*, **42**, 855–71.
5. Sandler, G. (1979). Costs of unnecessary tests. *British Medical Journal*, **2**, 21–4.
6. Hampton, J.R. *et al.* (1975). Relative contribution of history-taking, physical examination and laboratory investigations to diagnosis and management of medical outpatients. *British Medical Journal*, **2**, 486–9.
7. Fletcher, C. (1980). Listening and talking to patients, III. The Exposition. *British Medical Journal*, **2**, 994–6.
8. Enelow, A.J. and Swisher, S.N. (1986). *Interviewing and patient care*, 3rd edn. Oxford University Press, Oxford.
9. Cartwright, A. (1964). *Human relations and hospital care*. Routledge & Kegan Paul, London.
10. Dunkelmans, H. (1979). Patients' knowledge of their condition and treatment: how it might be improved. *British Medical Journal*, **2**, 311.
11. Hawkins, C. (1979). Patient's reactions to their investigations. *British Medical Journal*, **2**, 638–40.
12. Parkin, D.M. (1976). Survey of the success of communication between hospital staff and patients. *Public Health*, **90**, 203–9.
13. Reynolds, M. (1978). No news is bad news: patients' views about communication in hospital. *British Medical Journal*, **1**, 1673.
14. Ley, P. (1983). In *Doctor–patient communication* (eds. D. Pendleton and J. Hasler), pp. 89–107. Academic Press, London.
15. McNamara, M. (1974). Talking with patients: some problems met by medical students. *British Journal of Medical Education*, **8**, 17–23.
16. Firth-Cozens, J. (1987). Emotional distress in junior house-officers. *British Medical Journal*, **295**, 533–36.
17. Flexner, A. (1910). *Medical education in the U.S.A. and Canada. A report for the Carnegie Foundation for the Advancement of Teaching*, Bull. No. 4. Updike, Boston, Massachusetts; reprinted (1972) Arno Press.

18. Asher, R. (1972). *Richard Asher talking sense*, p. 170. Pitman Medical, London.

19. Meadows, R. (1977). Munchausen syndrome by proxy: the hinterland of child abuse. *Lancet*, **2**, 343–5.

20. Maguire, P. (1985). Barriers to the psychological care of the dying. *British Medical Journal*, **291**, 1711.

21. Morris, D. (1978). *Manwatching. A field guide to human behaviour.* Panther Books, London.

22. Maguire, G.P. and Rutter, D.R. (1976). In *Communication between doctors and patients* (ed. A.E. Bennett). Oxford University Press, Oxford.

23. Macartney, F.J. (1987). Diagnostic logic. *British Medical Journal*, **295**, 1325–33.

24. Barrows, H.S. (1973). *Problem-based learning in medicine*, Educational Monograph No. 4. McMaster University, Hamilton, Ontario.

25. Elstein, A.S. *et al.* (1978). *Medical problem-solving: an analysis of clinical reasoning.* Harvard University Press, Cambridge, Massachusetts.

26. Barrows, H.S. *et al.* (1978). *An analysis of the clinical methods of medical students and physicians.* McMaster University, Hamilton, Ontario.

27. Campbell, E.J.M. (1976). Basic science, science and medical education. *Lancet*, **1**, 134–6.

28. Campbell, E.J.M. (1976). Clinical science and medical education. *Clinical Science and Molecular Medicine*, **51**, 1–7.

29. De Dombal, F.T. *et al.* (1972). Computer-aided diagnosis of acute abdominal pain. *British Medical Journal*, **2**, 9–13.

30. De Dombal, F.T. *et al.* (1974). Human and computer-aided diagnosis of abdominal pain. *British Medical Journal*, **2**, 376–80.

31. Warner, H.R., Toronto, A.F., Veasy, L.G., and Stephenson, R.S. (1961). A mathematical approach to medical diagnosis: application to congenital heart disease. *Journal of the American Medical Association*, **177**, 177–83.

32. (a) Edelwich, J. and Brodsky, A. (1980). *Burn-out: stages of disillusionment in the helping professions.* Human Sciences Press, New York.
    (b) Roberts, G.A. (1986). Burn-out; psycho-babble or valuable concept? *British Journal of Hospital Medicine*, **36**, 194.

33. Patients Association (1982). *Self help and the patient.* A directory of national organisations concerned with particular diseases and handicaps. Patients Association. London.

34. (a) Todd, J. *et al.* (1982). *Someone to talk to; a directory of self-help groups and support services in the community.* Thames TV in association with the Mental Health Foundation, London.
    (b) The *Coping with* series (1985). Chambers, London.
    (c) The *Overcoming common problems* series. (1985). Sheldon Press.

35. Morell, D.C. *et al.* (1986). The "five-minute" consultation: effect of

time-constraint on clinical content and patient satisfaction. *British Medical Journal*, **292**, 870–73.

36. Roland, M.O. *et al.* (1986). The "five-minute" consultation: effect of time constraint on verbal communication. *British Medical Journal*, **292**, 874–6.

37. Eimeri, T.S. and Pearson, R.J.C. (1966). Working time in general practice: how general practitioners use their time. *British Medical Journal*, **2**, 1549–54.

38. Stott, N.C.H. and Davis, R.H. (1979). The exceptional potential in each primary care consultation. *Journal of the Royal College of General Practitioners*, **29**, 201–5.

39. Hinton, J.M. (1972). *Dying*, 2nd edn. Penguin Books, London. [see also *British Medical Journal*, (1980), **281**, 1328].

40. Kubler-Ross, E. (1970). *On death and dying.* Macmillan, New York.

41. Lewis, E. (1976). The management of stillbirth—coping with an unreality. *Lancet*, **2**, 619.

42. Bourne, S. (1968). The psychological effects of stillbirths on women and their doctors. *Journal of the Royal College of General Practitioners*, **16**, 103.

43. Black, J. (1987). Broaden your mind about death and bereavement in certain ethnic groups in Britain. *British Medical Journal*, **295**, 536–9.

44. Health Education Council. (1981). *The loss of your baby.* [in cooperation with the National Association for Mental Health and the National Stillbirth Study Group].

45. Leroy, M. (1988). *Miscarriage.* Macdonald Optima, London.

46. Jones, R.H. (1983). The use of chaperones by general practitioners. *Journal of the Royal College of General Practitioners*, **33**, 25.

47. Van Beukesom, J.A.H. (1973). In *Anxiety factors in comprehensive patient care* (ed. W.L. Rees), pp. 26–31. Excerpta Medica, Amsterdam.

48. Buckman, R. (1984). Breaking bad news. *British Medical Journal*, **288**, 597.

49. Ley, P. (1982). Satisfaction, compliance and communication. *British Journal of Clinical Psychology*, **21**, 241–54.

50. Korsch, B.M. and Negretti, V.F. (1972). Doctor–patient communication. *Scientific American*, **227** (No. 2), 66–71.

51. Blos, P. (1967). The second individuation phase of adolescence. In *Psychoanalytic study of the child*, Vol. 22. International University Press, New York.

52. Evans, J. (1982). *Adolescent and pre-adolescent psychiatry.* Academic Press, London.

53. Coleman, J.C. (1980). *The nature of adolescence.* Methuen, London.

54. Offer, D. and Offer, J. (1975). Three developmental routes through adolescence. In *Adolescent psychiatry*, Vol. IV (eds. S.C. Feinstein and P.L. Giovacchini). Jason Aronson, New York.

55. Green, R. (1985). Atypical psycho-sexual development. *Child and*

adolescent psychiatry: modern approach, 2nd edn (eds. M. Rutter and L. Hersov). Blackwell Scientific, Oxford.

56. Erikson, E.H. (1950). *Childhood and society*. Norton, New York.

57. Rutter, M., Maughan, B., Mortimore, P., Ounston, J., and Smith, A. (1979). *Fifteen thousand hours: Secondary schools and their effect on children*. Open Books, London.

58. Weatherley, D. (1964). Self-perceived rate of physical maturation and personality in late adolescence. *Child Development*, **35**, 1107–210.

59. Will, D. and Wrate, R.M. (1985). *Integrated family therapy: a problem-centred psychodynamic approach*. Tavistock Publications, London.

60. Cox, A., Holbrook, D., and Rutter, M. (1981). Psychiatric interviewing techniques. VI. Experimental study: eliciting feelings. *British Journal of Psychiatry*, **139**, 144–52.

61. Hawton, K., Osborn, M., O'Grady, J., and Cole, D. (1982). Adolescents who take overdoses: their characteristics, problems and contacts with helping agencies. *British Journal of Psychiatry*, **140**, 118–23.

62. Mrazek, P.B. and Bentovim, A. (1981). Incest and the dysfunctional family system. In *Sexually abused children and their families* (eds. P.B. Mrazek and C.H. Kempe). Pergamon Press, London.

63. Morrison, J., Roberts, J., and Will, D. (1987). Twenty myths that justify not investigating child sexual abuse. *Social Work Today*, July 20.

64. Jaemmet, A. (1981). The anorexic stance. *Journal of Adolescence*, **4**, 113–19.

65. Minuchin, S. (1974). *Families and family therapy*. Tavistock Publications, London.

66. Hawkes, C.H. (1974). Communicating with the patient—an example drawn from neurology. *British Journal of Medical Education*, **8**, 57–63.

67. Littlewood, R. and Lipsedge, M. (1985). Culture-bound syndromes. In *Recent advances in clinical psychiatry* (ed. K. Granville-Grossman), p. 105. Churchill Livingstone, Edinburgh.

68. Rosenfield, M. and Maine, D. (1985). Maternal mortality: a neglected tragedy. *Lancet*, **2**, 83.

69. British Medical Association. (1986). Report of the Board of Science working party on alternative therapy. *British Medical Journal*, **292**, 1407.

70. Poole, A.D. and Sanson-Fisher, R.W. (1979). Understanding the patient: a neglected aspect of medical education. *Social Sciences and Medicine*, **13A**, 37–43.

71. Helfer, R.E. and Ealy, K.F. (1972). Observation of paediatric interviewing skills. *American Journal of Diseases in Children*, **123**, 556–60.

72. Arluke, E. (1980). Roundsmanship: inherent control on a medical teaching round. *Social Sciences and Medicine*, **14**, 297–302.

73. Steele, S.J. and Morton, D.J.B. (1978). The ward round. *Lancet*, **2**, 85–6.

74. Afsal Mir, M. *et al.* (1986). Video and audio-tapes for teaching history-taking. *Medical Education,* **20,** 102–8.
75. Van Ments, M. (1983). *The effective use of role-play. A handbook for teachers and trainers.* Kegan Page, London.
76. Balint, M. (1957). *The doctor, his patient and the illness.* Pitman, London.
77. *Physicians for the twentyfirst century.* The GPEP Report. (1984). Association of American Medical Colleges, Washington, D.C.

Index